Managing Crisis and Risk in Mental Health Nursing

Edited by Tony Ryan

First published in 1999 by:
Stanley Thornes (Publishers) Ltd

Reprinted in 2001 by:
Nelson Thornes Ltd
Delta Place
27 Bath Road
CHELTENHAM
GL53 7TH
United Kingdom

04 05 / 10 9 8 7 6 5 4

A catalogue record for this book is available from the British Library

ISBN 0 7487 3336 1

Page make-up by Acorn Bookwork

Printed & bound in Great Britain
by Antony Rowe Ltd, Eastbourne

CONTENTS

CONTRIBUTORS

Keith Cash
Keith is Professor of Nursing at Leeds Metropolitan University and Director of the Centre for the Analysis of Nursing Practice. This is a joint venture between the University and Leeds Community and Mental Health NHS Trust and has a broad research programme into the assessment and management of risk and need in community nursing. He has worked as a mental health nurse in Britain and North America. He is currently researching the way that community mental health nurses construct risk and how these conceptions affect the management of their caseloads.

Mike Doyle
Mike is currently Risk Management Co-ordinator for the Mental Health Services of Salford where he has responsibility for co-ordinating clinical and non-clinical approaches to the management of risk. Previously, he worked as a forensic community mental health nurse and is co-chair of the RCN Forensic Community Mental Health Special Interest Group. He is actively involved in delivering training on risk management and has a particular interest in clinical risk assessment and management of harm to others from people with a mental disorder.

Jim Duckworth
Jim has been assessing and treating sex offenders since 1982. He is responsible for supervising staff who are key workers to sex offenders at the Edenfield Centre as well as having his own caseload. He is co-therapist with Pauline England for two groups within the community treatment programme for men who have sexually abused children. With Maeve Murphy and Pauline, he has won awards for innovative work with sex offenders.

Steven D. Edwards
Steven worked in the NHS for over eight years before leaving to study philosophy at the University of Manchester. He has written a number of well-received books including *Relativism, Conceptual Schemes and Categorical Frameworks* (1990), *Externalism in the Philosophy of Mind* (1994), *Nursing Ethics: A Principle-Based Approach* (1996) and most recently has edited *Philosophical Issues in Nursing* (1998). He has also published many papers in academic journals. His present research interests include philosophy of the body, philosophical aspects of disability and the philosophy of nursing. He is currently employed as a lecturer in the Centre for Philosophy and Health Care, University of Wales, Swansea.

Pauline England
Pauline has been working in the field of forensic mental health since 1988 and has five years' experience of groupwork with men who have sexually abused children. Pauline co-ordinates the community treatment programme for men who have

sexually abused children, based at the North West Regional Forensic Mental Health Service, and has a wealth of experience in this work. With Maeve Murphy and Jim Duckworth, she has lectured all over the country on assessing and treating sex offenders. Pauline also works with adult survivors of child sexual abuse, many of whom she sees in her clinic at a local women's prison.

Richard Gray

Richard has worked at the Maudsley Hospital in South London since 1993. He has worked as a research nurse and been involved in a number of projects including clinical trials of novel antipsychotic medications. He currently works with Professor Kevin Gournay as tutor-practitioner at the Institute of Psychiatry where he is establishing a medication management programme for mental health professionals.

Helen Hally

Helen has over 20 years of nursing experience within the NHS. Since 1984 she has worked with a variety of health authorities and trusts across London, usually with a strong community focus. She was Chair of the Community Psychiatric Nurses Association from 1987 to 1990. Since then she has been involved in several independent reviews and public inquiries. In April 1998 she moved from her post as Executive Nurse Director and Director of Adult Mental Health with Lewisham and Guy's Mental Health NHS Trust to her current post as Nursing Director for the State Hospital Board for Scotland.

Frank Hanily

Frank currently works as a primary care mental health team leader in the Ribblesdale Total Purchasing Project and is Associate Consultant with King's College Centre for Mental Health Services Development. He has held a number of senior clinical and management positions in Leeds and Salford and has specialist expertise in cognitive behavioural psychotherapy. His interests include mental health law, policy formulation, the management of change and staff training in the development of community services.

Martin Hird

Martin is currently employed by the Leeds Community and Mental Health Trust working as a clinical team leader. Most of his nursing career has been spent working as a community mental health nurse. His interest in the development of ethically informed relationships with service users has led to his current research study exploring service users' experiences of their screening assessments when performed by nurses.

Maeve Murphy

Maeve is currently working as a nurse practitioner and a forensic community mental health nurse at the Edenfield Centre in Manchester. She has been working with sex offenders for six years and currently co-facilitates a group for men who have sexually abused children. Maeve is a trained psychosexual counsellor and has been involved in the counselling of people with a variety of sexual or relationship difficulties. She is involved in the supervision of other professionals working in the psychosexual field at a local and national level. Maeve has a keen interest in education and has lectured on this subject all over the country. She is a visiting lecturer at the University of Central Lancashire.

Paul Needham

Paul is a senior lecturer in health care studies at Thames Valley University in London where he teaches mental health at diploma and first degree levels. Paul trained as a nurse in Salisbury and entered teaching after a 15-year career in mental health nursing, latterly as a manager and clinical specialist. He gained his honours degree in education at the Southbank University in 1992 and his masters degree in mental health interventions at Middlesex University in 1996. Paul has a number of research interests relating to the care of severely mentally ill people.

Tony Ryan

Tony worked in a number of nursing roles in the NHS for 10 years before joining the mental health charity Turning Point in 1992 where he worked until 2000 as area manager. He now works as Service Development Manager and Research Fellow at the North West Mental Health Development Centre based in Manchester. He has published work on nursing practice, nursing management, perceived risk and mental health. Tony completed his doctorate at Lancaster University examining risk perceptions in mental health and the strategies employed by users and carers for dealing with mental health risks.

Siobhan Sharkey

Siobhan received her PhD in anthropology in 1989 from the University of East Anglia. She trained as a mental health nurse at this time and specialized in rehabilitation and enduring mental illness after registration. In the last five years she has held posts as research and development co-ordinator and research/ practitioner. Siobhan is currently Senior Lecturer in Mental Health at Bournemouth University. Her research interests include risk assessment and management in relation to enduring mental illness.

Ann Stockford

Ann trained as a probation officer and is the manager of Turning Point's Gwydir Project in Cambridge which supports mentally disordered offenders in their own accommodation. She has a particular interest in the community provision of services for mentally disordered offenders.

Barry Thirkettle ·

Barry is a research fellow at the Centre for the Analysis of Nursing Practice in Leeds. Before joining CANP, as well as working in a variety of mental health nursing settings, Barry was a clinical coding author for the NHS Centre for

Coding and Classification and field worker for mental health nursing on the UK-wide Nursing, Midwifery and Health Visiting Teams Project. Barry's research interests include CPN caseload management, adolescents' risk perceptions and health-related behaviour and the use of routinely collected data for research.

Peter Wright
Peter is a psychiatric nurse and qualified social worker. He has a range of practitioner and managerial experience in the statutory and voluntary sectors and currently manages Alfred Minto House, a community-based forensic mental health project for Turning Point in Nottingham.

ACKNOWLEDGEMENTS

I would like to thank the following people who have supported this book in one way or another: Janis Williamson, Keith Soothill, David Edwards, Bernie Eddisford, Barbara Hatfield, Mike Smith, Ian Smith, Malcolm Rae, Jane Mann and Tony Wayte. I would also like to thank the contributors who made my job much easier than I was told it would be!

I am also indebted to Turning Point for actively supporting me throughout this venture.

Tony Ryan

The authors and publishers would also like to thank Carfax Publishing Limited, PO Box 25, Abingdon, Oxfordshire, OX14 3UE for permission to reproduce Table 4.1, p.47; and Her Majesty's Stationery Office for permission to reproduce Table 3.3, p.30.

DISCLAIMER

In many of the chapters in this volume case studies are used to illustrate crisis and risk management situations that can arise in mental health nursing. While these case studies are based on experience, the people they describe are fictitious.

FOREWORD

Mental health nurses continue to occupy a central role in the provision of mental health services and this serves as a testimony to their continued ability to offer professional, skilled and sensitive care to people distressed and distracted by the problems of mental illness. There are always exceptions and a number of inquiries into service failures have highlighted shortcomings by nurses as well as other staff. However, evidence for the central role played by mental health nurses is overwhelming and without their skilled presence services would fail alarmingly. In sustaining this central role, mental health nurses have adapted to and often led major changes in the orientation of care (hospital to community), their own education, changes in government policy and the quite proper demands to involve people and their families who use services.

Feeling comfortable about innovative ways of thinking in the delivery of mental health services and being able to utilize new techniques in assessment and intervention mean mental health nurses must attend continuously to their understanding of new ideas and service developments. The nature, definition and operational consequences of crisis and risks are vital elements of professional practice and this book makes a timely and essential contribution to our understanding and responsibilities as mental health professionals.

I welcome this book. As the reader will see, it offers a comprehensive review of the context in which difficult decision making must take place, offers commentary and strategic help in crisis and risk management and debates those special circumstances which surround the management of crisis and risk. To say that crisis and risk management is an emotive and difficult subject is to state the obvious. This book deals with situations which are faced by most mental health nurses day in and day out. Until now, many of the skills and assessment strategies which nurses use to assess and manage risk and crisis have been poorly described and articulated; this book has done both these things with success. Indeed, the authors take an extra step in both describing and dealing purposefully with difficult clinical decisions and complement this by helpful and supportive information which, while not condoning clinical failure, allows it to be debated carefully and dispassionately.

The book is produced at a time when the government has declared a sustained investment in mental health services and has highlighted the deficiencies of present-day community care. New services are to be developed for the most difficult and challenging patients and this will obviously require 'knowledgeable doers' to provide services to those most in need and at risk. As usual, mental health nurses will be in the front line of service provision. This book will help them and other mental health professionals to provide a safer and more sensitive service that the public both reasonably expects and deserves.

Professor Tony Butterworth CBE, FRCN
University of Manchester 1998

INTRODUCTION

In drawing on the expertise of nurses in clinical practice, management and academia, it is hoped that this collection of papers will help to clarify key questions for nurses and other mental health professionals charged with balancing issues relating to crisis and risk in mental health care.

The concepts of crisis and risk are important in modern mental health care, particularly given the publicity that surrounds events where something has gone wrong. Not only does such publicity fuel negative and misleading images of people who experience mental health problems, it also reduces confidence in those who are charged with managing such risks. The way that risk has been defined to date in mental health has been largely to do with physical harm to self or others. Nevertheless, there is an increasing acknowledgement that people with mental health needs experience a number of other risks, for example loss of dignity through stigma. Therefore, the book also considers issues from the position of those who are thought to face or pose particular risks: the mental health service user.

The principal aim of this book is to provide a guide for mental health nurses and professionals ancillary to nursing to define, assess and manage crises and risks in relation to people with a range of mental health needs. This collection of papers explores the concepts of crisis and risk in relation to context, decision making and clinical practice. Naturally, what constitutes a crisis or risk differs given a particular set of circumstances and the individuals involved. Hence, throughout the text risk is defined as it relates to particular contextual, decision-making and clinical circumstances. Therefore, various definitions of risk are used in this book. However, crisis is defined as the point at which an unwanted risk outcome is about to materialize.

Part One examines the contextual and decision-making issues that arise in crisis and risk management. Current knowledge concerning how people understand the concept of risk is examined from individual, group and cultural perspectives. This illustrates that risk is a dynamic concept which continually changes as a result of experience and circumstance. By contrast, the way in which risks have gone wrong in mental health care is also discussed and the lessons to be learned are highlighted. Additionally, legal, policy and organizational frameworks are addressed. Part Two examines questions of clinical nursing practice in relation to a number of areas. Key issues are considered in relation to both hospital and community settings with definitions of risk being particular to the context and location. Part Three considers questions that have caused controversy and debate in the past within the field of mental health. It examines issues that underlie justifications for making interventions on behalf of service users and how users can be involved in the process of risk management. The role of psychopharmacology and its appropriateness in the management of crisis and risk are discussed, as are the methods available to nurses to improve their decision-making when dealing with crisis and risk situations.

Those who work within modern mental health care recognize that we can never live in a risk-free world and there will be occasions where unwanted risk outcomes occur. Similarly, those who have experience of mental health problems are increasingly, and correctly, being seen as active and informed participants who are encouraged to take a proactive role in addressing their needs. Hopefully, this book will go some way to ensuring that mental health nurses are able to assist service users to deal successfully with crisis and risk situations or make decisions on their behalf that are in their best interest and the interests of those closest to them.

Tony Ryan

PART ONE

CONTEXTUAL AND DECISION-MAKING ISSUES IN CRISIS AND RISK MANAGEMENT

1 RISK KNOWLEDGE AND MENTAL HEALTH NURSING

Tony Ryan

INTRODUCTION

The concept of risk has become an important theme within society at the end of the millennium. Currently, knowledge about how the concept of risk relates to mental health is still in its infancy. Consequently, it is worth exploring how risk is understood in other areas to see if anything can be learned which might improve understanding in mental health care. In this chapter, four areas of risk are examined which have a direct relevance to the field of mental health and its notion of risk. *Cognitive psychology* has produced a wealth of knowledge about how people perceive risk and react to risk perceptions. *Cultural theory* has examined how risk perceptions and reactions are influenced by groups. *Sociologists* have examined how society and organizations respond to risk while the discipline of *law* has developed ways of deterring risk taking and spreading the cost of risk. What is known about risk in these areas has a direct relevance for how risk is understood in the field of mental health. Therefore, it is essential knowledge for mental health nurses wishing to understand how the concept of risk relates to their field of work.

ON THE NATURE OF CRISIS AND RISK

Crisis, like risk, is ill defined in mental health care. For the purposes of this work, crisis is regarded as the point at which an undesired risk outcome becomes highly likely or has occurred. Risk management is about preventing future harms where time is available to plan interventions and management strategies. Crisis is concerned with the management of such risks when they are about to result in negative consequences. Crisis is often best defined by service users as this engages people at the time of greatest vulnerability. It is also client centred and empowering for service users.

Risks are now more evident than ever in society and are related to increased knowledge about new technologies and ways of living. Innovations in the technological and social sciences have led to an increased knowledge of the risks associated with new developments. Some of this knowledge raises awareness of risks that have always existed, such as the increased risk of lung cancer associated with smoking cigarettes. Therefore, we may know more about something and, as a result, make a better informed decision about the associated risks. This, however, does not necessarily reduce the risks to which we are exposed; it merely heightens our awareness of such risks. There may also be risks we are not aware of at the time of making risk decisions but this does not mean they do not exist.

Renn (1992) suggests that there are two diverse ends of a spectrum of risk. At one end is the view that risk is an objective property which comes from an event or activity and is measurable. At this end of the spectrum, risks can be graded in terms of their probability and implications. Resources can then be allocated to dealing with those at the top of the list first, in order that a systematic approach be implemented to deal with risks in a society. At the opposite end of the spectrum is the notion that risk is a cultural phenomenon which cannot be graded because of the social values and contexts present in risk events or activities.

Statistical measures of risk, such as the number of road deaths per annum or the incidence of suicide in a particular geographical area, serve a purpose in that they can provide a basis for encouraging particular desirable behaviours or health promotion activities. However, risk assessment of this form does not account for the qualitative aspect of risk. Such assessments frequently omit to take account of the changes in quality of life which occur as a result of the road death of a family breadwinner or the effects upon the partner of a person who commits suicide.

In exploring risk as if it has form, we can give it boundaries. The *form* of risk is often in quantity. For example, the risk of developing a particular mental illness may be more accurately predicted through applying knowledge about factors which add to the risk: family history, geographical area, personal circumstances and so forth. When this is done, we can go on to calculate problems associated with the risk and thereby transform it into something tangible and measurable. As we shall see later, the scientific objectification of risk does not allow for the qualitative nature of the risk experience which is socially and culturally constructed.

For Luhmann (1993), risk accommodates a plurality of distinctions within one concept. Every decision and indecision, action and inaction contains a risk even if it is only the risk of not grasping opportunities which may have been advantageous. Distinctions are made by observers, between what they see and what they do not see. Risk is a phenomenon of multiple contingency which produces different perspectives in different observers. Risk is not only about physical harm or financial loss but can cover less observable or tangible things such as reputation and dignity.

Krimsky (1992) suggests that there are greater concerns within society about fatalities and injuries from events concentrated in time or space than from events which are widely dispersed across time or geography. The former group are often seen as catastrophes, the latter as non-catastrophes, with greater efforts put into reducing the frequency of catastrophes. This is exemplified currently in mental health by comparing efforts to reduce homicides by people with mental health problems with the efforts applied to reducing media misrepresentation of people with mental health needs. The risk of physical harm is far more tangible than the risk of stigmatization.

THE PSYCHOLOGY OF RISK PERCEPTION

Early exploration into the psychology of risk perception took place in the area of judged fatality. Lichtenstein and colleagues (1978) found that people overestimate the frequency of deaths which were typically vivid or imaginable, such as those caused by tornadoes or road traffic accidents, and underestimate those which are less imaginable, such as from botulism or diabetes. A suggested reason for this is the *availability heuristic*, a method people use to evaluate individual risk situations (Kahneman *et al.*, 1982). The issue being explored is matched with information most readily available and recalled. Therefore, the more *available* the information, the more likely the event will be viewed as going to happen. Hence, shortly after a high-publicity disaster, such as a plane crash or a homicide by a mentally ill person, the perception of risk associated with the event will increase. This is the case even though in real terms the true possibility of it recurring is no greater than before the event first happened. Even when the event is known to have a low statistical probability of recurrence the risk perception will be greater than if the event had not occurred. Several studies demonstrate the availability heuristic hypothesis as central to how people perceive risks (Combs & Slovic, 1979; Tversky & Kahneman, 1973). It is worth noting that the concept of risk means more to people than just fatalities and in some cases, the risk may seem worse than death, such as paraplegia or brain damage (British Medical Association, 1987).

Slovic (1987) notes that lay people's perceptions of risk have strong qualitative and subjective aspects. By comparison, 'expert' perceptions are less qualitative and more likely to be related to quantitative features such as the number of deaths that would occur from a particular risk. Many other findings have been generated from risk perception studies. Lay people have problems in determining probabilistic information on risks (Slovic *et al.*, 1980). The way that risks are presented to people influences how they are perceived; for example, whether or not the risk is presented as positive or negative can affect the results generated (Kahneman & Tversky, 1984). From the early work in this area, it has been widely acknowledged that risk perception involves a number of qualitative features such as the voluntary and involuntary nature of the risk (Starr, 1969). Green & Brown (1979) note a distinction between two dimensions: the individual and societal nature of risks, for example snakebite as opposed to nuclear radiation.

Limited work has been undertaken in the area of perceived risk concerned with mental health. Nevertheless, it has been shown that public perception changes immediately after a high-profile incident but this reduces to original levels of concern over time (Appleby & Wessely, 1988). A further finding is that women consistently regard a wide range of risks associated with mental illnesses to be greater than men, irrespective of position as user, carer, professional or member of the public (Ryan, 1998).

This work is useful in understanding the nature of risk but there are issues that need to be borne in mind when reviewing the contribution of cognitive psychology. First, it is difficult to reduce risk to a single measurable concept since social and cultural patterns in society affect the very way in which risk is perceived. In addition, much of the psychological literature has focused upon the individual rather than the group. The aggregation of individual responses does not necessarily take account of group influences on the individual and their perceptions.

CULTURAL THEORY AND RISK

The perceiver of risk is rarely isolated and lives within social and cultural systems that affect beliefs and behaviours regarding risks. In this sense risks are socially and culturally structured and authenticated or legitimized. Societies and institutions fashion the way risks are perceived by the individual. These systems also shape what is of value to the society and what is not. This includes which risks are to be legitimized and significant and which are to be disregarded (Douglas, 1986). This can be seen in the moral panic associated with the issue of caring for mentally ill people in community settings (Muijen, 1995).

According to Douglas & Wildavsky (1982) risk perception is a process which can only be understood by recognizing underlying social, cultural and moral characteristics which are responsible for overstatement or understatement of a particular risk. They argue that people's concerns in relation to risks are really an expression of social solidarity. From this perspective it becomes easier to understand why some risks are disregarded despite being more hazardous; for example, the widespread concern about homicides by mentally ill people compared with the risk of death by tuberculosis which is given far less attention yet kills greater numbers of people.

Within this model risk and risk perceptions are not defined by nature but by social and cultural factors; consequently they are dynamic and constantly changing. Risk means different things to different people and has developed beyond something purely positivistic to be measured by experts in terms of the probability of loss since it has many qualitative aspects to it.

It has been suggetsed that 'Preferences for risk ... can be explained by the function those preferences serve for an individual's way of life' (Thompson et al., 1990, p.63). Risks reflect the distribution of power and status in society. The impoverished are likely to be exposed to a larger number of risks than those who are financially better off. Those who live in areas of high deprivation are subject to higher rates of crime, unemployment and poor health than people in more affluent areas (Alaszewski et al., 1997). Hence there will always be differences in risk perception between policymakers and other stakeholders in relation to mental illness.

People identify with and take part in various social groupings. Risks which are significant to the individual are those which affect the various groupings in which they associate. Viewpoints on risk are therefore not consistent as they are exposed to cultural forces which are continually changing and causing the perception of risk to be dynamic. Various attitudes and beliefs about the nature of risk are generated from within the group and are then assimilated by the individual members. Individuals may hold differing views within the group but the group itself will be a dominant force in determining how they articulate and act in relation to risk. Douglas (1982) refers to this as *cultural bias*.

Cultural theory puts forward the view that a person's cultural bias is linked to the extent to which they are incorporated into groups and the extent to which the interactions are conducted according to rules rather than negotiated *ad hoc* (Royal

Society, 1992). This perspective suggests that the choice of risks for attention within a society are not the result of predetermined factors of a biological or psychological nature within the individual. Instead, they are chosen by group members as a method of protecting the way that the group lives. Risks therefore are a forensic resource which can be used to apply blame to other groups for adopting a differing lifestyle, a lifestyle which may threaten the group (Douglas, 1992, 1993). Examples of this in mental health can be seen in differences between user movements or service providers and the local communities who protest against new mental health facilities being developed in their area.

Despite the influence of the group on risk perceptions, it needs to be recognized that most people do not exist within a single social grouping. As people move from group to group, their risk perceptions will be affected accordingly. Therefore risk perceptions adjust to changing influences experienced by the individual.

SOCIAL FEATURES OF RISK

Beck (1992) suggests that in postmodern society we face the problem of the distribution of risks and hazards produced through the process of modernization. He argues that there are five factors which pertain to risk (Box 1.1). While Beck wrote about the *risk society* from a perspective which mainly examined technological risk, it is easy to see how his thesis can be applied directly to the field of mental health.

Within any risk situation there are three groups: decision makers, those affected and beneficiaries. It is not possible to divide these into heterogeneous groups as much depends upon the context in which each decision is made and the perspective

---

Box 1.1

Beck's thesis on risk

1 Risks are socially constructed. They are accentuated or attenuated through social institutions such as the media or professional groups. Experts are rarely non-scientific.

2 Risk positions develop as risks grow. Not all risks are equally distributed, nor are they always geographically contained.

3 With risk comes potential exploitation. Risk knowledge carries financial opportunities. Lack of knowledge on risk issues brings financial and other dangers.

4 Risk knowledge has a political significance which can mean that some risks are played down whilst others are highlighted for attention.

5 Socially recognized risks develop a political dimension particularly if it is desirable for a risk to be removed. Where those in positions of power choose a risk eradication option in responding to a risk, there will be losers.

---

from which it is viewed. In any situation, an individual may be in all three of these categories or there may be two or more different individuals or groups concerned with a particular risk. For example, at a section 117 meeting users, professionals and carers may be present and may fall into a number of these three categories. Professionals are decision makers but are also affected if things go wrong and are beneficiaries if they do not. Users and carers are rarely true decision makers in such fora but are affected by the decisions and therefore can be beneficiaries.

In wider society it is not always possible for individuals to make every risk decision that affects them. Therefore many decisions are made by small numbers of people, the consequences of which may affect large numbers, for example, mental health professionals. In making such decisions, Luhmann (1993) argues, there are two perspectives and subsequent paths which can be followed. First, the perspective of the decision maker looking to improve decisions through the use of complicated calculations or elaborate assessment techniques, which in mental health has led to a proliferation of risk assessment methods. The second perspective is that of the affected, where appeasing communication is frequently given by the decision makers to those affected. Examples of this can often be seen in the communication between mental health professionals and service users or carers and also in government responses to public concern.

In the case of organizations, attempts are often made to control the decision making through rational and bureaucratic action, yet perfectly rational decisions are impossible. Even though a decision maker may decide on the basis of a large amount of information they can never be certain that the information they use is everything that exists. There is always the possibility that something has been overlooked or is not known about a risk. Although deciding to wait until further information becomes available may be an option, it is also a non-decision which in itself can have risks attached to it.

Luhmann (1993) suggests that in the case of organizations, every task is reduced to the level of a decision. Decisions are concatenated: one decision triggers another and so on until the product is finally arrived at. Within the organization this bureaucratic process reduces the possibility of individuals making unwanted decisions in isolation. It also provides, in theory at least, the opportunity to identify who made the decision which produced the undesired event.

Organizations tend to concentrate on probabilities and improbabilities when making risk decisions. Security is gained from numbers when taking risk decisions and also from who make up the numbers, as with multidisciplinary teams operating to mental health policy. Experts, consultants and people with experience combine to provide a greater illusion of safety and security. The effort invested supports the claim that all possible precautions are taken to avoid an unwanted event or disaster. Reassurance is the name of the game even if it is only an illusion. The constant checking and linking of subdecisions increases the sense of security. Where an unwanted event has occurred it is rarely viewed as predictable in any way, unless the predictability is associated with system failure. This can be seen in many of the recent homicide inquiries which have highlighted poor communication as system failure in the mental health system.

Where decisions lead to an undesired event, organizations are frequently unable to learn from the unfortunate circumstance. A favoured option of bureaucratic organizations is to identify a person whom they can charge as accountable. Scapegoating places the blame for the wrong risk decision with the individual rather than the organization and its methods of reaching decisions. Only recently have processes been investigated in mental health decision making through inquiries (Sheppard, 1995). Despite the welcome advance of having inquiries, such measures are open to the challenge of having little impact. They can merely allow organizations to be seen to be doing something as a response to risk events rather than actually adjusting the systems the organization has in place (Carson, 1996).

Where the focus is upon individuals, rather than the processes which allowed them to make the risk decision, this can encourage people to be risk averse. This is because taking a decision which results in an undesired outcome can mean loss of employment, which in most cases the individual values (Luhmann, 1993). Risk taking is an important part of mental health nursing but an emphasis on individuals rather than processes can lead to conservative practice (Ryan, 1994).

THE LEGAL INTERPRETATION OF RISK

Lowi (1993) claims that risk takers are necessary for the advancement of a society and that legal systems act as an intermediary on risk. Markets, including the health and social care market, contain risks which require rules and regulations to make them function effectively. The role of law is to create a balance between risk takers, the prospective risks they bring to the society and the individuals who may be injured in some way because of the actions of the risk takers. A relevant example here could be a community where people are to be resettled from a regional secure unit.

From a legal perspective, risk is used as a shorthand term for the *foreseeability test* which relates to a standard of care and can form the basis for the imposition of strict liability (Hepple & Matthews, 1991). Rogers (1989) suggests that there are two elements which combine to determine the magnitude of a risk. These are the likelihood that an injury will transpire and the seriousness of the damage that is risked. Carson (1988) argues that risks are situations where action or inaction has been chosen in order to achieve a desired outcome with the knowledge that harm could occur.

Liability for professional activities is now expanding as concern increases about professional safety standards. In law, there has been a move away from socially acceptable levels of risk toward using individual cases as examples to force improved safety measures and reduce risks. Hence the steady increase in the UK recently of claims against health professionals for negligence (Tingle, 1997) although this has not been considerable in the mental health field. Large damages are awarded with this in mind and also with deterrent and punitive elements, for example as with car safety, vaccines and serious medical errors (Handmer & Penning-Rowsell, 1990). In mental health this was exemplified by the Tarasoff case in the United States where confidentiality was maintained and a death resulted (see Tarasoff v. Regents of the University of California, 1976). New test cases are brought forward all the time which claim that a particular risk was not adequately communicated at the time a person was exposed to it. Furthermore, the concept of strict liability can apply in tort law where risks are not known at the time products are used, as with anxiolytic medicines and subsequent dependency.

Contract law and tort law

The law of contract allows people to agree terms for the allocation of risks. The contract is an agreement reached between two parties to control specific aspects of the future and the associated risks (Lowi, 1993). Tortious law is based on case law and therefore constantly changing as it is influenced by the thinking of the day. Tort law allocates risks *ex post facto* where the individuals were not in a position to enter a contract because they could not bargain or because the costs involved in contracting exceeded the resources available to do so.

The major form of liability in tort law is that of fault liability which is based upon negligence or the intention to cause injury. Even so, there are situations where the concept of strict liability applies and can arise without fault being present or proven. In general, tort law requires the plaintiff to demonstrate that the defendant caused the injury. The problem of motive is generally inconsequential in connection with liability; irrespective of whether the motive is good or bad, the liability will remain the same. Unlawful conduct with honest motive will result in liability just as lawful activity with dishonourable motive will not result in liability.

Legal protection against risk

There are a range of defences which an individual can employ to avoid liability. *Formal consent* may have been obtained, as with a medical operation. There are many other areas where consent is said to have been obtained even though it has not been formally agreed and put in writing such as 'a fair blow in a boxing match, an inoculation, a welcomed embrace ... because the plaintiff consents to them' (Rogers, 1989, p.683). Consent must be of an informed nature where the plaintiff has full knowledge of the circumstances with which they are agreeing and has chosen this option after being made aware of alternative courses of action.

Liability may be avoided where it can be proved that an *accident* occurred even though reasonable care was exercised. The defence of *necessity* can be used, for example where a person assists someone who is unconscious and requires medical help (Rogers, 1989). Such defences to avoid liability are responses which occur after the event. The chief form of avoiding liability prior to the risk event is through insurance.

Coleman (1992) points out that insurance spreads rather than reduces risk, leaving tort law to allocate the costs of accidents and claims. Priest (1993) argues that a principle of modern law is to reduce accident rates through allocating the expense of actions in such a manner that it is more cost effective to take loss-avoiding action than it is to pay for the injuries caused. From this perspective it can be seen that insurance is a form of risk management which allows for a blurring of individual responsibility.

Both of these methods of avoiding liability are now coming increasingly to the forefront of mental health care in many countries. At present within the UK it is possible for NHS trusts to spread the risk of claims through the NHS pooling scheme (Clinical Negligence Scheme for Trusts, 1996). Additionally employers, and increasingly individual practitioners, insure against professional negligence as a means of protecting themselves against the future.

RISK ISSUES FOR MENTAL HEALTH NURSES

The concept of risk is difficult to define in a number of fields and particularly mental health nursing. However work on risk in other areas can help to clarify risk issues in mental health nursing. How does the experience of risk in other fields relate to mental health nursing? Clearly, there are many ways in which individual perceptions of risk are affected. Availability of information, how information is presented, the vividness of negative risk outcomes and how much control the person feels they have over the risk have all been shown to impact on individual risk perceptions. Compounding these factors is the influence that groups have upon individuals in the way they perceive and respond to risk. Furthermore, the type, style and aim of the organization where nurses work will also influence how they perceive and deal with risk. There are also clear messages from a legal position that provide a framework for nurses who deal with risk in their work.

Much of this work, as with risk work generally in mental health, regards risk as something negative and to be avoided. However, it is important for mental health nurses to keep an eye on the wider picture. While risk work is an important area of mental health nursing, it should not be regarded as purely a negative force. A central tenet of current practice is that of empowering people who use mental health services to take control of their lives and illnesses. To achieve this nurses need to be aware that risks come in a range of different forms and for the most part are concerned with risk to service users rather than other people (for a review, see Ryan, 1996). It should be remembered that risk work can be a positive experience for service users and nurses, particularly when taking therapeutic risks aimed at empowering the user (Ryan, 1993).

REFERENCES

Alaszewski, A., Walsh, M., Manthorpe, J. & Harrison, L. (1997) Managing risk in the city: the role of welfare professionals in managing risks arising from vulnerable individuals in cities. *Health and Place.* 3:1, 15–23.

Appleby, L. & Wessely, S. (1988) Public attitudes to mental illness: the influence of the Hungerford massacre. *Medicine, Science and the Law.* 28:4, 291–296.

Beck, U. (1992) *Risk Society: Towards a New Modernity.* London: Sage.

BMA Professional and Scientific Division (1987) *Living with Risk: The British Medical Association Guide.* Chichester: John Wiley.

Carson, D. (1988) Risk-taking policies. *Journal of Social Welfare Law*. 328–332.

Carson, D. (1996) Structural problems, perspectives and solutions. In: J. Peay (ed) *Inquiries After Homicide*. London: Duckworth, pp. 120–146.

Clinical Negligence Scheme for Trusts (1996) *Risk Management, Standards and Procedures: Manual of Guidance*. Bristol: CNST.

Coleman, J.L. (1992) *Risks and Wrongs*. Cambridge: Cambridge University Press.

Combs, B. & Slovic, P. (1979) Causes of death: biased newspaper coverage and biased judgements. *Journalism Quarterly*. 56, 837–843.

Douglas, M. (1982) *Essays in the Sociology of Perception*. London: Routledge & Kegan Paul.

Douglas, M. (1986) *Risk Acceptability According to the Social Sciences*. London: Routledge & Kegan Paul.

Douglas, M. (1992) *Risk and Blame*. London: Routledge.

Douglas, M. (1993) Risk as a forensic resource. In: E.J. Burger (ed) *Risk*. Ann Arbor, Michigan: University of Michigan Press, pp. 1–16.

Douglas, M. & Wildavsky, A. (1982) *Risk and Culture: An Essay on the Selection of Technological and Environmental Dangers*. Berkeley: University of California Press.

Green, C.H. & Brown, R.A. (1979) Counting lives. *Journal of Occupational Accidents*. 2, 55–70.

Handmer, J. & Penning-Rowsell, E. (1990) Is success achievable? In: J. Handmer & E. Penning-Rowsell (eds) *Hazards and the Communication of Risk*. Aldershot: Gower Technical, pp. 311–326.

Hepple, B.A. & Matthews, M.H. (1991) *Tort: Cases and Materials*, 4th edn. London: Butterworth.

Kahneman, D. & Tversky, A. (1984) Choices, values and frames. *American Psychologist*. 39:4, 341–350.

Kahneman, D., Slovic, P. & Tversky, A. (eds) (1982) *Judgement Under Uncertainty: Heuristics and Biases*. Cambridge: Cambridge University Press.

Krimsky, S. (1992) The role of theory in risk studies. In: S. Krimsky & D. Golding (eds) *Social Theories of Risk*. Westport, Connecticut: Prager Press, pp. 3–22.

Lichtenstein, S., Slovic, P., Fischhoff, B., Layman, M. & Combs, B. (1978) Judged frequency of lethal events. *Journal of Experimental Psychology*. 4, 551–578.

Lowi, T.J. (1993) Risks and rights in the history of American governments. In: E.J. Burger (ed) *Risk*. Ann Arbor, Michigan: University of Michigan Press, pp. 17–40.

Luhmann, N. (1993) *Risk: A Sociological Theory*. New York: de Gruyter.

Muijen, M. (1995) Scare in the community. Part five: Care of mentally ill people. *Community Care*. 7–13 September (supplement), i–viii.

Priest, G.L. (1993) The new legal structure of risk control. In: E.J. Burger (ed) *Risk*. Ann Arbor, Michigan: University of Michigan Press, pp. 207–227.

Renn, O. (1992) Concepts of risk: a classification. In: S. Krimsky & D. Golding (eds) *Social Theories of Risk*. Westport, Connecticut: Prager Press, pp. 3–22.

Rogers, W.V.H. (1989) *Winfield and Jolowicz on Tort*, 13th edn. London: Sweet & Maxwell.

Royal Society (1992) *Risk: Analysis, Perception and Management*. London: Royal Society Study Group.

Ryan, T. (1993) Therapeutic risks in mental health nursing. *Nursing Standard*. 7:24, 29–31.

Ryan, T. (1994) The risk business. *Nursing Management*. 1:6, 9–11.

Ryan, T. (1996) Risk management and people with mental health problems. In: H. Kemshall & J. Pritchard (eds) *Good Practice in Risk Assessment and Risk Management*, Volume 1. London, Jessica Kingsley Publications, pp. 93–108.

Ryan, T. (1998) Perceived risks associated with mental illness: beyond homicide and suicide. *Social Science and Medicine*. 46:2, 287–297.

Sheppard, D. (1995) *Learning the Lessons: Mental Health Inquiry Reports Published Between 1969–1994 and their Recommendations for Improving Practice*. London: Zito Trust.

Slovic, P. (1987) Perception of risk. *Science*. 236, 280–285.

Slovic, P., Fischhoff, B. & Lichtenstein, S. (1980) Facts and fears: understanding perceived risk. In: R.C. Schwing & W.A. Albers (eds) *Societal Risk Assessment: How Safe is Safe Enough?* New York: Plenum Press.

Starr, C. (1969) Social benefits versus technological risk. *Science*. 165, 1232–1238.

Tarasoff v. Regents of the University of California (1976) California Reports 14, 551 P.2d 334.

Thompson, M., Ellis, R. & Wildavsky, A. (1990) *Cultural Theory*. Boulder, Colorado: Westview.

Tingle, J. (1997) Healthcare litigation: working towards a culture change. *British Journal of Nursing*. 6:1, 56–57.

Tversky, A. & Kahneman, D. (1973) Availability: a heuristic for judging frequency and probability. *Cognitive Psychology*. 4, 207–232.

2 INQUIRIES INTO THE CARE OF MENTALLY ILL PEOPLE: THE LESSONS

Helen Hally

INTRODUCTION

Things go wrong. In any sphere of activity where people are working together to provide a service to other people, errors, unexpected occurrences, confusions, miscommunications and skills deficits may all conspire to produce unwelcome situations. Health care is not immune to these processes. Over recent years there have been several high-profile examples of things going very wrong in general health care. The failures in the cervical and breast-screening programmes in Kent and Canterbury, Bristol and Exeter affected thousands of women and, quite rightly, high-level inquiries were conducted into the circumstances that lead to such failures.

In mental health the inquiry culture is well established. Untoward or serious incidents involving mental health service users will now routinely trigger some degree of inquiry, ranging from a local internal review, through board level scrutiny, to an extensive public inquiry in the full glare of the media spotlights.

In this chapter I intend to describe the path that has lead us to this point and to give an overview of the inquiry process, before reflecting on what we can learn from such inquiries.

THE HISTORY OF INQUIRIES

In reviewing the path taken to this point I will resist the temptation to go back to 1632 and the report of the Privy Council inquiry into conditions at Bethlem Hospital which, according to David Sheppard (1995) in his introduction to the first edition of *Learning the Lessons*, was the first recorded inquiry.

I will begin instead in 1969. The Ely Hospital Inquiry (1969) was significant for many reasons. It was really the first major inquiry into a whole hospital system. Although it was triggered by and had as its focus several specific allegations made against certain staff, it was the hospital culture that came under scrutiny. The allegations were made by a nursing assistant and this made Ely the first in a series of inquiries running through the 1960s and 1970s that were prompted by junior staff drawing attention to their concerns about the conduct of more senior staff. The allegations were brought into the public domain by the *News of the World* newspaper, establishing a still active tradition of the media's involvement in mental health campaigning.

This inquiry was also significant in that it prompted the then Health and Social Services Secretary, Richard Crossman, to establish the Hospital Advisory Service, whose initial function was to act as the eyes and ears of the Health Secretary, to ensure that never again could a health care system decline into such an abusive and dysfunctional state. In 1976 the Hospital Advisory Service became the NHS Health Advisory Service with a broadened remit to include community services.

Hard on the heels of Ely came the 1971 Farleigh Hospital Inquiry and, in 1972, the Whittingham Inquiry. Both of them were shameful indictments of the malpractices, ranging from petty tyranny to manslaughter, that could develop in what were largely closed institutions.

Over the next 13 years, a further 20 inquiry reports were published. One of these related to a fatal attack on a member of staff by a service user. All the others followed allegations of either clinical or, less frequently, administrative malpractice. The services that came under scrutiny were either mental health or learning disability inpatient settings and were predominantly of the county asylum type. The reports make chilling reading and are powerful advocates for the hospital closure programme that, somewhat paradoxically, is in some quarters blamed for the events addressed by the next wave of inquiries.

In 1987 a panel was set up to:

- inquire into the management of arrangements for the care and aftercare of Sharon Campbell;
- consider the adequacy of these arrangements;
- report to the Secretary of State and to make recommendations, on the basis of their findings, on any measure or practices which might provide improvements in identifying the needs of mentally disordered people and in the quality of care for those living in the community and the support for staff working with them. (Spokes *et al.*, 1988, p.45).

Sharon Campbell was an outpatient when she fatally attacked her former social worker in her office at Bexley Hospital. Today, an inquiry would have followed swiftly. Then, although the killing took place in July 1984, it was not until March 1987 that an inquiry was set up and even then it was only because of the continued pressure for such an inquiry from the social worker's father, a doctor.

The influence of the Sharon Campbell inquiry was significant. It led to the introduction of the Care Programme Approach (CPA) and also demonstrated the legitimacy of enquiring into the care management of people even if they were no longer in receipt of services at the time of the incident.

In 1990 two inquiry reports were published: one into the death of an inpatient at the hands of another inpatient; the other into the death of an inpatient following the administration of medication. Up until 1991, reports had largely dealt with real or perceived dysfunctional organizations. Occasionally, they had addressed the deaths of fellow service users or members of staff. In 1991, three reports were published into circumstances that were to become all too familiar over the next six years. The names Barratt, Findley and Kirkman have not entered the mental health lexicon in the way that Campbell and Clunis have done, but their actions and the subsequent reports have significance.

Carol Barratt, supported by her mother, took her discharge against medical advice from a mental health unit. Two days later she stabbed and killed an 11-year-old girl. Stephen Findley also took his discharge against medical advice and five days later stabbed and killed a 67-year-old man. Both of the victims were strangers to their attackers. At the time this was a very rare occurrence but it served to fuel fears about the failures of care in the community. The next attack on a stranger took place less than a year after the publication of these reports, to be followed three months later by the fatal stabbing of Jonathan Zito by Christopher Clunis.

These events and the subsequent high-profile reporting and campaigning reinforced the public perception that people with mental health problems were a threat to us all. In reality, of the 45 inquiry reports published between 1990 and 1997, only seven have been initiated as a result of an attack on a stranger. In the same period, there have been 19 reports dealing with fatal attacks on relatives.

The first of these was the report published in 1991 into the care of Kim Kirkman. As part of a planned rehabilitation programme, Kim Kirkman had a day's leave from his mental health unit. Whilst on leave he killed his fiancee before returning to the unit in the evening. The killing by a service user of a relative may or may not have been rare as an event; however, at that time it was certainly rare as the subject of an inquiry. There were no such reports in 1992 or 1993. There was one in each of the two following years. However, in 1996 there were reports from eight such inquiries and the same number in 1997. Over this same period, reports of inquiries into apparent dysfunctional systems, the hospital scandals that were the main focus of early inquiries, became far less frequent. There were four in 1992, including a thoroughly damning report on Ashworth Special Hospital, one in 1993, two in 1994 and one in 1996 (details of these reports can be found in Sheppard, 1996). There were no such reports in 1997 or 1998, however, the Fallon Inquiry published another damning report on Ashworth in January, 1999.

From this it can be seen that there has been a significant shift in the focus of inquiries since 1969. Earlier work was hospital focused; latterly, the focus has been on community provision. Earlier inquiries looked at things done to service users; later inquiries have explored things done by service users. However, when inquiries have been well conducted they have all given attention to what it was in the way that services were conceptualized, organized and delivered that made system failure and individual tragedy possible. It is from this that recommendations about change on a local and national basis flow. These recommendations are the justification of the inquiry process. Inquiries should not be about identifying individuals who are to blame. There are management and disciplinary processes and, in extreme circumstances, criminal justice channels that are appropriate for this. Inquiries should address the broader factors that contribute to a system's failure and the changes needed to reduce the chance of repetition.

THE INQUIRY PROCESS

Before looking at what we can learn from inquiry reports, I would like to explore briefly the ways in which inquiries may be established and how they are likely to conducted. All that follows is somewhat speculative because as yet there is no standardized approach to inquiry procedure. The most detailed central guidance comes under *Health Service Guidance, HSG(94)27*. This guidance, and it is guidance not instruction, recommends that following a homicide involving someone, either as victim or perpetrator, who has had previous contact with the specialist mental health services, an independent inquiry should be set up and a published report should be available to the public. The variation in the interpretation of this guidance has led some inquiry reports to comment on the inquiry process and to make recommendations about how they should be conducted (Greenwell *et al.*, 1997; Lingham *et al.*, 1996; Ritchie *et al.*, 1994).

However, in broad terms, a panel is convened and chaired by someone with a legal background. Panel members, usually two or three, are recruited, with backgrounds that equip them to deal authoritatively with the matters under review. For example, if nursing practice were under scrutiny, it would be usual to have a nurse on the panel. This is, however, by no means a hard and fast rule.

While the panel is being assembled, the terms of reference are defined and agreed. The panel then agrees its method of working. An early decision has to be taken on whether the hearings should be held in public or private. Neither is a comfortable option, either for staff or for the relatives of the victim or the perpetrator. Private hearings may help staff to feel less exposed while giving evidence, but it deprives them of the opportunity to acclimatize themselves to the process before being called. Neither do they have a clear context for the evidence they are giving. They do not know what has gone before them and what has influenced the line of inquiry adopted by the panel. For relatives, it is difficult to imagine how they could be satisfied with the thoroughness of the inquiry unless they are party to the collection of evidence. There is both the potential for healing and for great pain in hearing, at length, details of the circumstances that led to their particular tragedy. On this issue, I tend to side with Sir Louis Blom-Cooper who advocates open hearings with the twin justification, that 'sunlight is the best of disinfectants' and that open justice 'keeps the judge, while trying, under trial' (quoted by Justice Brandeis, p.9, and Jeremy Bentham, p.16, in Blom-Cooper *et al.*, 1995).

As soon as an inquiry has been commissioned, all relevant and available documentation is gathered. Tracking down, indexing, copying, reading and annotating the clinical records along with summaries of records held by other agencies, witness statements and other varied material is a considerable task. The thoroughness and orderliness at this stage will have significant bearing on the quality of the inquiry. The panel members will meet to discuss the material they have read. Further documentation may be requested at this stage, and indeed, throughout the proceedings. A list of people who will be required to give evidence will be agreed and letters sent out to each individual informing them of this and the areas that their evidence should address. This will usually include a request for a written statement prior to the hearing.

At the hearings, witnesses may be led through their evidence by members of the inquiry panel. This is now by far the most usual approach. Sometimes, however, a counsel to the inquiry will be appointed who, under the direction of the panel, will ask the majority of the questions, with panel members asking for clarification or expansion on occasions. Such an approach has a tendency to introduce an almost adversarial atmosphere, which is perhaps not the most effective way of arriving at a true account of events. In the larger scale, more complex inquiries, as in the current Ashworth Inquiry, such an approach is perhaps highly beneficial.

Usually there is a full transcript made of the oral evidence. This is invaluable when the panel retire to write their report. Good practice dictates that all witnesses are given a copy of the transcript of their evidence and the opportunity to correct any errors or clarify any ambiguous areas. This is not, however, a universal practice.

The next stage is the writing of the report. Again, approaches vary. Some reports are written by a secretary to the inquiry, who submits drafts to the panel for approval. Some reports are written by the inquiry chair and again approved by the panel. Other reports are produced by all members of the panel, each writing designated sections and coming together to edit the pieces into a seamless whole. Each approach has its merits, but they all take time.

Time is one of the major concerns about the inquiry process. From the incident to the publication of the inquiry report may take anything from six months to two years. For an incident involving a homicide that is not followed by the suicide of the perpetrator, 14 months is about the average. That is a very long time for relatives to live with the uncertainty and stress inevitably involved in any inquiry. It is also an extremely long time for services and staff to be kept under a shadow. Anything that can shorten this period without compromising the thoroughness of the inquiry must be of benefit to all concerned.

The length of time that inquiries take from incident to report is one major concern. There are others. The high and sometimes excessive costs of inquiries, the lack of standardization in approach and the lack of any central mechanism for assessing, endorsing (or otherwise) and reflecting in policy the many and varied recommendations that come from these inquiries have given rise to much speculation about alternatives to our current system.

At one stage it looked as though the Health Advisory Service might have been well placed to take on a role outlined in the *Report of the Inquiry into the Treatment and Care of Raymond Sinclair* (Lingham *et al.*, 1996), Recommendation 12:

(i)   *A panel should be set up to supervise inquiries commissioned under Health Service Guidelines HSG(94)27.*

(ii)   *The panel should be responsible for creating a register of those suitably qualified, both professionally and in their interpersonal skills, to sit on such inquiries.*

(iii) *It should also publish a recommended form of procedure and additional guidance designed to reduce delay and the stress caused to witnesses, particularly the relatives of the deceased and other victims, and to encourage cost effectiveness.*

With the 1996 review of the Health Advisory Service and the subsequent recasting of the organization as a research and consultancy body, this opportunity was lost.

December 1997 saw the launch of a new White Paper: *The New NHS: Modern*
• *Dependable.* Among its proposals is the establishment of a Commission for Health Improvement. This body is described thus:

> *As a statutory body, at arms length from Government, the new Commission will offer an independent guarantee that local systems to monitor, assure and improve quality are in place ... the Commission will be able to intervene on the direction of the Secretary of State ... the Commission will both investigate and identify the source of the problem, and work with the organization on lasting remedies ... The Commission will have a membership drawn from the professions, NHS, academic and patient representatives ...*
>
> (Department of Health [DoH], 1997, pp. 7.13, 7,14)

Perhaps in this, a reworked and extended Health Advisory Service, there is again the potential for establishing the sort of standardization and rigor that is currently a fundamental flaw of the inquiry system.

So far, I have commented only on the external, independent inquiry process. There are many other forms, depending on the complexity and perceived seriousness of the situation under review. Following a serious incident, and the criteria for defining an occurrence as such vary considerably from organization to organization, a board-level or equivalent decision should be taken about the appropriate category of review. This may be internal at service level, internal at board level, internal at board level with external support, external reporting to the board or external and public. Trusts and other mental health organizations should have their own serious incident policy that sets out the criteria for each level of review and details the process to be followed. The South Devon Healthcare Trust Report (1994) recommended that 'Incidents should be kept under constant review by an Incident Review Committee established for the mental health service; and Mental Health Act Managers should be encouraged to review quarterly reports by the Committee to the Board of the Trust' (Blom-Cooper *et al.*, 1994, p.85). The flaws associated with public inquiries are also present, though perhaps to a lesser degree, in all other levels of inquiry. They consume considerable resources, take time to complete and therefore place all concerned under considerable stress for a prolonged period, generate recommendations that may or may not get integrated into practice and are immensely variable in method, thoroughness and competence.

The current system may be flawed. However, there is much to be learned from the inquiry process and the resulting reports. One of the challenges is to distil from the myriad recommendations, many of which are only locally specific, many of which are contradictory, those elements that can provide a solid base for policy and practice development. Matt Muijen (1997) has pointed out the apparent paradox that 'The recommendations of the earlier inquiries into community care have been so much more influential than those in later reports' (p.18), despite the fact that reports are being produced at a far greater rate now than has ever been the case. Increased activity does not seem to have resulted in a greater store of collective understanding, nor, with the depressing regularity that the same system failures are described in report after report, does there appear to have been much impact on practice.

LEARNING FROM INQUIRIES

The Zito Trust, in *Learning the Lessons* (Sheppard, 1996), attempts to analyse recommendations from inquiries published between 1985 and 1996. This takes 68 pages. I am not going to attempt anything on that scale. Instead, I will highlight a few areas that I believe have particular relevance for nurses.

First, though, a few words about what will not be found in inquiry reports. A defensiveness has crept into mental health clinical practice based on the belief that if any course of action taken by a clinician is followed by an untoward incident, a modern-day witch-hunt will ensue with the sole purpose of identifying and blaming the clinician. For example, an informal inpatient has an agreed care plan that includes weekend leave if judged well enough to go by the ward manager. The ward manager assesses the service user, documents that assessment and leave is granted. The service user subsequently takes an overdose. Such an incident should be reviewed, at a level determined by the trust policy. Such a review will be a difficult experience for all involved. However, no censure should be attached to the ward manager if the process agreed within the care plan was followed.

Similarly, a clinician who decides, following a full examination and assessment, not to admit someone who presents at casualty will not be criticized if the person subsequently kills themself, so long as the assessment, the reasons for not admitting and the proposed treatment plan are all fully and contemporaneously documented. I know of no inquiry report where a clinician is blamed if his or her risk assessment proves to be inaccurate.

This is not to suggest that individuals are never criticized, nor that the absence of criticism renders the experience of being involved in a serious incident and the subsequent inquiry painless. However, clinicians who can demonstrate that their actions were considered, that they were acting within local, national and professional guidelines, assuming responsibility appropriate to their competence, making the best use of all available information and communicating effectively with all relevant stakeholders have nothing to fear from the inquiry process. This message is not made explicit within inquiry reports; it can be inferred from the criticisms and recommendations that are made when these circumstances do not prevail. However, I believe that it is an important message to get across to all clinicians working in the field of mental health. No one is expected to predict the unpredictable; we are all expected to anticipate and plan for that which can be predicted. We cannot eliminate risk, but we can manage it.

Risk information

Recent inquiry reports have highlighted some of the areas in which practice can and must be improved in order to manage risk more effectively.

'Risk assessment is concerned with making a prediction. That is, making an estimate of the likelihood that a particular event will take place' (Harbour *et al.*, 1996, p.69). The cornerstone of making any estimate about the likelihood of a particular event taking place is information. When making a significant decision based on the predictability of an event, many sources of information may be consulted. Before going hill walking, any serious hiker will want to know what sort of weather to expect. Sources of this information may include previous personal experience, examination of the cloud formation, direct contact with the local meteorological station and consultation with other local walkers. This information will be considered and result in a decision that either the risk factors are too great to proceed or that the risk factors can be managed through adequate preparation.

This is a process with which we are all familiar. Decision making based on information about the probability of certain events is a central part of our daily lives. However, inquiry after inquiry reveals how crucial decisions are based on inadequate or inaccurate information that has adversely influenced the estimation risk.

Rarely, the information is sought but is not forthcoming. More frequently, inadequate attempts are made to gather all available information, or available information, particularly the views of carers, is disregarded, or undue reliance is placed upon information that has become distorted over time through a 'Chinese whispers' process.

Neither the full history of domestic violence, nor Evan B's full criminal record appear to have been made available. In the absence of this information and in the absence of evidence of mental illness the decision to discharge Evan B from hospital was understandable. If the information had been available then it is possible that he might have been detained in hospital to allow for an assessment by the forensic service.

(Bromley Health Authority, 1997, p.10)

4.5.9 In our opinion, the events as they unfolded in the hospital were the next major failing in the system. Firstly, none of the staff took the opportunity to seek information on what was going on at home from Marcus, who was with Gilbert when he was admitted, neither did they telephone Mrs Kopernik-Steckel for her views or tell her what was happening.

4.5.10 Dr Lawrence failed to make the home situation or the level of danger clear to the hospital staff. He was not proactive in providing any information for them.

(Greenwell *et al.*, 1997, p.21)

If close relatives, including Andrew's next of kin, had difficulty in getting their voices heard, then it is perhaps not surprising that other friends and supporters had even greater difficulty in generating a response to their cries for help.

(Blom-Cooper *et al.*, 1995, p.145)

We have shown that it is insufficient to rely on discharge summaries, which in themselves may be conflicting, and from which it is impossible to judge how thorough the writer has been in their compilation. Sometimes it seems that, when the history reaches a point of overwhelming complexity, the past history is enigmatically summarized, "see past discharge summaries", all of which contain one or two similar trite phrases meant to sum up the wisdom gleaned over many years. There is no alternative to the painstaking methodical review of past notes.

(Blom-Cooper *et al.*, 1995, p.180)

The importance of gathering detailed and accurate information from all available sources cannot be overestimated. Failure to do so fundamentally weakens any subsequent assessment and care planning. The recommendations relating to this particular aspect of care are legion (Sheppard, 1995, p.50), but sadly, the lessons are still not being learned.

Risk communication

Gathering information is not an end in itself. For effective care delivery, information has to be gathered, processed, recorded and used to inform decisions about care. It must also be shared. It is in this area of information sharing that shortcomings are identified again and again.

There is scarcely a single published inquiry report that does not describe basic failures in ensuring that everyone involved in providing care to an individual knew what was going on. The communication gulfs have on occasion come from a mistaken belief that withholding information was in the service user's best interest. 'However, he told us that if they pointed him in the direction of another hostel they would not disclose his violent history, because that would jeopardize his place' (Ritchie *et al.*, 1994, p.46).

More frequently, these gulfs, which can be between agencies, between disciplines or between statutory and voluntary sectors, result from a basic lack of understanding of the crucial nature of full and effective communication in the delivery of care to people with complex needs. The roots of this may lie in mistaken beliefs about the precedence of confidentiality over all other considerations. They may lie in the unidisciplinary training tradition in this country; nurses have nursing information that they share with nurses, but they don't share it with social workers or doctors. Such a position is patently absurd and with the advent of integrated clinical records for all disciplines and interagency working becoming the norm, there is room for optimism that this position may improve.

The lack of appreciation of the need for good communication may also stem from a prevailing health service culture that perceives that clinical work is being swamped by time-consuming bureaucratic imperatives. It is still possible to hear clinicians of all disciplines railing against the CPA because of how it gets in the way of clinical work. The CPA *is* clinical work. Good communication with others involved in the complex care arrangements for an individual is clinical work. As countless inquiries have demonstrated, we ignore this at our peril and individuals who are considered to have been wanting in their approach to communication will be criticized.

Risk recording

A further aspect of clinical information management that comes in for much comment is record keeping. In her foreword to *Keeping the Records Straight*, Yvonne Moores writes:

> *The fundamental importance of record keeping as a foundation of care cannot be emphasized too strongly. Accurate, complete and up-to-date records represent a vital component of high quality care ... Some of the messages and real life examples outlined in the course are deliberately shocking – particularly when the potential consequences of poor records are examined.*
>
> (National Health Service Training Directorate [NHSTD], 1993)

The responsibilities for nurses are made explicit in the United Kingdom Central Council's (1993) publication *Standards for Records and Record Keeping*. Nevertheless, for some reason that is difficult to understand, there seems to be a universal poverty in the mental health records of our clients. Generally, they are badly organized with information being filed, if filed at all, out of sequence. Multiple records without crossreferencing are frequent, even within the same agency.

> *The Trust should undertake a project to consolidate and amalgamate the various sources of information, particularly separate sets of case notes, about patients attending different facilities.*
>
> (Hughes *et al.*, 1995, p.29)

> *One step that could and should have been taken as a matter of urgency, was the abandonment of separate professional notes, and the development of multidisciplinary records. At the same time as integrating professional notes into a single record, attention should be paid to integrating hospital and community records. The ideal to aim for is a single mental health record for each patient, irrespective of where they are treated, or by whom.*
>
> (Blom-Cooper *et al.*, 1995, p.140)

Duplications and omissions abound. Handwritten entries fall into two main categories: either they are almost illegible yet contain important information or they are easy to read with no useful content. Usually, I consider a defensive stance unhelpful to the development and delivery of high-quality care. In relation to clinical records, I take a slightly different position. The situation is so dire that I would urge every clinician to be fully conscious each time they make an entry in the notes that if something untoward occurs in relation to that client, then that entry will come under full and thorough scrutiny. Standing in a coroner's court or before a panel of inquiry being questioned on an immaculately written record is daunting enough; to have to defend the standard of record that is all too frequently presented could be, at best, highly embarrassing.

Individual and organizational responsibilities

Responsibility for developing best practice in all the areas outlined above lies partly with the individual and partly with the organization within which the individual works. Sharing that responsibility does not dilute it. As stated in the *Code of Professional Conduct* (UKCC, 1993), nurses are personally accountable for their practice. This does not change, even if the organization has responsibilities to ensure that staff have at their disposal the systems, support and resources to deliver best practice. The interface between individual and organizational responsibility comes to the fore around the issue of supervision.

There is a duty on the individual to practise safely; safety in clinical work cannot be guaranteed in the absence of high-quality, appropriate supervision. In mental health, clinical work without supervision is like solo pot-holing without a rope. The organization has a responsibility to ensure that systems are in place to deliver the required supervision, but its absence does not absolve the individual from personal responsibility.

Several recent inquiry reports have given considerable attention to the issue of supervision. The recommendations from *Working in Partnership* that 'new training initiatives aimed at developing clinical supervision skills in senior clinical nurses are devised. We also recommend that newly qualified nurses and nursing students receive preparation in what to expect from clinical supervision' (DoH, 1994, p.45) have been fully endorsed and both the *Viner Report* (Harbour *et al.*, 1996) and *The Falling Shadow* (Blom-Cooper *et al.*, 1995) have further recommended the development of a mandatory supervision system for all disciplines at all grades.

The supervision issue links back directly to information management. As discussed earlier, information management has several component parts. It covers information gathering, and we have seen how inquiries have repeatedly revealed inadequacies in this area. It covers information recording, and again this is an area of glaring deficits. It covers information sharing and the inability or unwillingness of staff to pass on essential information is repeatedly identified as a major factor in the tragedies under investigation.

The role of supervision in information management is in information processing. Supervision is a way of ensuring that the relationship between the clinician and service user does not unduly influence objective risk assessment. We all tend to make allowances for people we feel close to. Similarly, if we have difficulty establishing a relationship with someone, we may see them as a greater threat than someone with whom we have built up rapport. Through supervision, any subjective bias can be identified and therefore taken into account when assessing risk. Without this, the risk assessment and therefore risk management process is flawed and, inevitably, further inquiries will follow.

CONCLUSION

What can we learn from inquiries into the care of mentally ill people? Since 1969, the focus of inquiries has shifted from an examination of organizations providing care for a large number of service users to an exploration of the experience of care and treatment for an individual person. Each serious incident has its own unique features, but common to all is the contribution made by inadequate information management. If we can learn to gather, process, record and share clinical information effectively and efficiently, then we will be making significant strides towards the sort of care that our clients, our colleagues and our community deserve. Serious incidents will still occur. Mental illness is a high-risk area but through managing information, we will be taking appropriate action to minimize that risk.

REFERENCES

Blom-Cooper, L., Hally, H. & Murphy, E. (1994) *Report to the South Devon Healthcare Trust*. Torquay: South Devon Healthcare Trust.

Blom-Cooper, L., Hally, H. & Murphy, E. (1995) *The Falling Shadow: One Patient's Mental Health Care 1978-1993*. London: Duckworth.

Bromley Health Authority (1997) *Report of the Independent Inquiry Team Following a Homicide by a Service User in April 1996*. Bromley: Bromley Health Authority.

Department of Health (1994) *Working in Partnership: A Collaborative Approach to Care*. London: HMSO.

Department of Health (1997) *The New NHS: Modern • Dependable*. London: The Stationary Office.

Greenwell, J., Procter, A. & Jones, A. (1997) *Report of the Inquiry into the Treatment and Care of Gilbert Kopernik-Steckel*. Croydon: Croydon Health Authority.

Harbour, A., Brunning, J., Bolter, L. & Hally, H. (1996) *The Report of an Independent Inquiry into the Circumstances Surrounding the Deaths of Robert and Muriel Viner*. Ferndown: Dorset Health Commission.

Hughes, J., Mason, L., Pinto, R. & Williams, P. (1995) *Report of the Independent Panel of Inquiry into the Circumstances Surrounding the Deaths of Ellen and Alan Boland*. London: North West London Mental Health NHS Trust.

Lingham, R., Candy, J. & Bray J. (1996) *Report of the Inquiry into the Treatment and Care of Raymond Sinclair*. Aylesford: West Kent Health Authority.

Muijen, M. (1997) Independent inquiries: why less is more. *Mental Health Practice*. 1:3, 18.

National Health Service Training Directorate (1993) *Keeping the Records Straight*. London: NHSTD.

Ritchie, J., Dick, D. & Lingham, R. (1994) *The Report of the Inquiry into the Care and Treatment of Christopher Clunis*. London: HMSO.

Sheppard, D. (1995) *Learning the Lessons*. London: Zito Trust.

Sheppard. D. (1996) *Learning the Lessons*, 2nd edn. London: Zito Trust.

Spokes, J., Pare, M. & Royle, G. (1988) *Report of the Committee of Inquiry into the Care and After-care of Miss Sharon Campbell*. London: HMSO.

United Kingdom Central Council (1993) *Code of Professional Conduct*. London: UKCC.

3 POLICY AND LEGISLATION IN THE MANAGEMENT OF CRISIS AND RISK

Frank Hanily

INTRODUCTION

Mental health policy has had an emphasis on developing community services over the past 30 years with the cumulative effects becoming more noticeable over the past 10 years. In the 1990s media attention has shifted from hospital inquiries to inquiries into care in the community (Muijen, 1996). One significant outcome of this has been a recognition of the importance of risk assessment and management in the care and treatment of mentally ill people.

Legislation is by far the most important single part of constitutional law, other forms being common law, conventions and constitutions and the law and custom of Parliament. Legislation can be both regulatory and enabling, as in the case of the Mental Health Act (1983) that applies to England and Wales. It sets the ground rules of what is permissible and what is not. Policy, on the other hand, is designed to guide and advise practice. In the mental health field, there are specific legislative influences such as the Mental Health Act (1983) and the recent amendment to it, the Mental Health (Patients in the Community) Act (1995). Policy initiatives specific to mental health include the Care Programme Approach (CPA) and the supervision register. One of the principal functions of legislation and policy is to manage risks associated with mental illness and enable crises to be managed safely for the benefit of those concerned. An example of this in risk assessment and management could be a compulsory admission to hospital for treatment where it is judged that a person is at significant risk of harming themselves or the public.

In mental health work, risk assessment and risk management are seen as ongoing and include such notions as *likelihood* and *potential*. For most professionals, and particularly mental health nurses, crisis has a narrow and specific definition. It is associated with a point in time where an immediate decision is required because of the acute nature of the situation. The mental health policy and legislation that covers risk and crisis issues can be found in the Mental Health Act (1983), the CPA, supervision registers and the Mental Health (Patients in the Community) Act (1995). These initiatives affect a number of stakeholders in the field of mental health (Table 3.1).

CURRENT ISSUES

The expectations of mentally ill people have changed greatly since the programme of deinstitutionalization began around 1955. This is now acknowledged in the *Patient's Charter* (Department of Health [DoH], 1997a). In the 1960s, once a

Table 3.1	Stakeholder	Interests and responsibilities
Risk stakeholders	Government	Providing services and caring for sick people. Protecting the public.
	Professionals	Delivering services. Protecting the public.
	Service users	Avoiding unnecessary detention. Accessing appropriate services for treatment.
	Carers	Supporting their relatives/significant others. Prevention of abuse.
	Public	Protection from harm. Accepting mentally ill people.

person was discharged from hospital, mental health services had no further responsibility so a mechanism of inquiry into community services was not necessary. This is no longer the case, as a large number of inquiries into the care of people in community settings over the last decade demonstrates.

In the 1990s, two-thirds of the mental health budget is accounted for by maintaining hospital beds (Audit Commission, 1994) which creates difficulties in the transfer of mental health services to community settings. The number of hospital beds has reduced from a high of approximately 150,000 in 1955 to 40,000 in 1994 (Audit Commission, 1994). One of the effects of this reduction in beds has been to raise the admission threshold for people with acute mental health problems. The remaining beds are often in poorly designed units built in district general hospitals which, coupled with the higher admission threshold, has led to an increase in violence (Lelliott *et al.*, 1995; Shah, 1993). There are accounts of a crisis in mental health beds in London and there are often occasions when all the mental health beds in the south of England are occupied (Lelliott *et al.*, 1995). Therapeutic interventions are difficult in such environments and there is a need for nurses to develop skills in treating the severely mentally ill person. Additionally, schizophrenia and major affective psychoses are often complicated by substance misuse, therefore needing hospital beds for much longer periods (Mental Health Act Commission, 1997). Further, this report highlighted the need for mental health nurses to update skills to reflect the current demands being placed on hospital beds.

There is a need to balance restrictive policies and legislation with adequate provision and support for mentally ill people who are most at risk and present the greatest danger to themselves and the general public. This chapter examines the development of recent policy and legislation and discusses the implications for mental health nurses.

THE MENTAL HEALTH ACT (1983)

The Mental Health Act (1983) remains the main body of regulation for the care and treatment of mentally ill people in England and Wales. Therefore, managers and practitioners should have a sound working knowledge of the legislation (DoH, 1996; DoH & Welsh Office, 1993). This is particularly true of mental health

Table 3.2

The role and responsibilities of mental health nurses in relation to the Mental Health Act 1983

Power/issue	Knowledge required
Detained people: sections 2, 3, 4 & 5(2)	• Check the documents are legally completed (e.g. each paper relates to the same person and is properly signed). Rectifiable mistakes (such as incorrectly spelt names) should be rectified within 14 days. • Ensure that mentally ill people are aware of and understand their rights and a leaflet is given about their detention. • Ensure that a letter and leaflet explaining detention are sent to the nearest relative. • Good practice would dictate that the nurse activates the appropriate community services (e.g. community mental health team).
Leave of absence: section 17	• Ensure that the form is completed correctly with a copy to the detained person and a further copy filed in their case notes. No-one should go on leave without a valid and correct section 17 form. • A person cannot be recalled from leave just for the purpose of detention and then granting immediate leave (Regina v. Hallstrom).
Renewal of section	• Renewal of section 3 commences when the doctor completes form 30. This normally takes place during the two months prior to the end of section 3 and comes into effect on the expiry of the previous section.
Consent to treatment (medication): section 58	• Three months after medication has first been administered the consultant psychiatrist must interview the person and obtain informed consent to treatment (three month rule). If not obtained a written *second opinion* must be obtained from a Mental Health Act Commission-approved doctor.
Consent to treatment (ECT)	• Form 38 should be completed by the responsible medical officer or second opinion appointed doctor where the person consents to treatment. This form should state the number of proposed applications of ECT. • Where valid consent is not obtained the responsible medical officer must comply with the requirements of section 58, which should be implemented as soon as possible.
Mental health review tribunal	• In the case of section 2, detained people must apply within 14 days. In the case of section 3, detained people can apply at any time. • Advise and help the person to apply for a tribunal. • Good practice suggests that the nurse should attend the tribunal with the detained person.
Mental Health Act Commission	• Ensure that detained people are aware of a visit by the Commission, if planned, or have opportunity to speak if unannounced. • Ensure that there is a private consultation room.

nurses given their central role in the care and treatment of mentally ill people in both hospital and community settings.

Most of the treatment under the Act takes place on hospital wards which are largely managed and staffed by nurses. Here, mental health nurses become involved in a range of essential activities; for instance, receiving documentation on people who are detained under the Act (*sectioned*), caring for and treating people and managing situations where detained people will not comply with treatment. Table 3.2 summarizes the key areas of responsibility for mental health nurses.

In community settings, mental health nurses have long been involved in the aftercare arrangements of mentally ill people (section 117) and vulnerable people (guardianship orders; section 7 and section 37). More recently, nurses have had a role under the Mental Health (Patients in the Community) Act (1995), which is discussed later in this chapter.

The Mental Health Act (1983) made clear the legal position of nurses by enacting section 5(4): nurses holding power. This section can be used to detain people who are in hospital and not already detained. Section 5(4) enables a nurse to use the holding power when it appears:

> *(a) that the patient is suffering from mental disorder to such a degree that it is necessary for his health or safety or for the protection of others for him to be immediately restrained from leaving the hospital; and*

> *(b) that it is not practicable to secure the immediate attention of a practitioner for the purposes of furnishing a report under section (2), that is a doctor is not available to assess and detain, if necessary, the patient under section 5(2).*

(Mental Health Act, 1983, p. 5)

The nurse invoking these powers must be a registered mental nurse or registered mental handicap nurse and it only applies to people already receiving treatment in hospital. The actions of the nurse are guided by the *Mental Health Act Code of Practice* (DoH & Welsh Office, 1993). Before using the power the nurse takes into consideration:

- the likely time of arrival of the doctor;

- the consequences for the person leaving immediately;

- known unpredictability and other relevant information available to the multidisciplinary team.

The person detained under section 5(4) has no right of appeal against the decision so adequate training and supervision are essential for nurses working in these settings, alongside the use of regular audit.

There has been a steady increase in the use of section 5(4) from 1053 in the year ending 31 March 1991 to 1401 in the year ending 31 March 1996 (DoH, 1997b). This is hardly surprising given the reduction in beds and increase in violence cited above. The emergency nature of the power is recognized as putting added anxiety and stress on both mentally ill people and staff involved (Ashmore, 1992). Nevertheless, it is acknowledged as an essential crisis management tool where there is no resident doctor (Cooper & Harper, 1992).

THE CARE PROGRAMME APPROACH (CPA)

Health authorities were required to introduce the CPA in 1991 (DoH, 1990). The CPA was further extended to incorporate risk work – risk to both the mentally ill person and the public (DoH, 1994). It now forms the cornerstone around which all mental health care is planned (DoH, 1996). In broad terms, anyone who is involved with specialist mental health services is entitled to be included in the CPA. It ensures that those who are especially vulnerable or who pose a risk in other ways due to a mental illness will receive appropriate mental health and social

---

Box 3.1

The elements of the CPA

1. Systematic multidisciplinary assessment of health and social care needs.
2. A written care plan agreed between relevant professionals, the person and main carers.
3. The allocation of a key worker to co-ordinate services.
4. Regular review of the person's progress and their continuing health and social care needs.

---

care in the community. Additionally, care management is provided by local authority social services departments. They have specific duties under the NHS and Community Care Act (1990) to assess the needs of the person for community care services, to formulate a plan and ensure its implementation. Care programming and care management are founded on the same principles and are closely linked. There are four basic elements to any care programme (see Box 3.1).

The CPA has not had an easy passage into mental health practice and did not work as intended when first introduced (DoH, 1993). There was widespread confusion about its meaning and its relation to the other changes in providing care for mentally ill people (Schneider, 1993), with poor co-operation between health authorities and social services departments highlighted (DoH, 1995). Consequently, the tiered CPA was introduced in *Building Bridges* (DoH, 1996) as a pragmatic step to address many of the problems arising.

Table 3.3

The tiered approach to the CPA

Level	Application
Minimal CPA	Applies to people with low support needs who are likely to remain stable. Commonly only one practitioner will be involved.
More complex CPA	The person is likely to need more than one type of service and/or their condition is less likely to remain stable. Several team members will be involved, including (almost certainly) a psychiatrist, social worker and mental health nurse. The care plan will be more complex, requiring interventions from several team members with careful attention being paid to the identification of the key worker.
Full, multidisciplinary CPA	This applies to people with severe mental illness, suffering from severe social dysfunction, whose needs are likely to be highly volatile or who represent a significant risk. Again, the process of identifying the key worker needs thorough discussion. In cases where the person presents a significant risk to themselves or others, the consultant psychiatrist, together with their colleagues, should consider whether inclusion on the supervision register is appropriate. Some services may choose to regard the supervision register as an additional *top tier* of the CPA.

(Source: Department of Health (1996). Crown Copyright material is reproduced with the permission of the Controller of Her Majesty's Stationery Office)

| CASE STUDY 3.1 | **THE ROLE OF THE MENTAL HEALTH NURSE IN THE CARE PROGRAMME APPROACH** |

John is 22 years old and was diagnosed as suffering from paranoid schizophrenia three years ago. He has never been willing to comply with medication regimes as he complained that they slowed him down and he disliked the extrapyramidal side-effects. He frequently misses outpatient appointments and appointments with his community nurse. He has never been admitted to hospital largely because of the support he has received from his family.

Five months ago, following a family dispute, John left home and moved into a social services hostel for young men. After a short period he moved to his own flat and has not maintained any links with his family. However, he has been in regular employment in a local supermarket on the meat counter and enjoys his work.

He missed a number of outpatient appointments and the nurse never seemed to be able to find him at home or work. Consequently, the mental health services had no contact with him for a period of six months until his employer got in touch with his GP expressing concern about a violent incident at work where John had threatened a colleague with a meat cleaver. After the nurse met with John it became clear that he was experiencing paranoid delusions and believed his colleague was plotting to harm him. Detention under the Mental Health Act (1983) for treatment was discussed as an option between the GP, nurse and psychiatrist but as John was willing to return to his parents' home and be treated there, this was not necessary. His condition quickly responded to medication and he also agreed to take a fortnightly depot injection. His community nurse initiated a care programme meeting to ensure that John continued to be supported. In preparation for this, John was assigned a social worker who undertook a full social needs assessment during which John stated that he was happy to remain in the family home indefinitely. The nurse accompanied John to meet with his employer and assist him to negotiate a return-to-work package.

At the care programme meeting John agreed that he should remain in the family home and return to work at the supermarket. The nurse was appointed as keyworker as it was deemed that she was best placed to co-ordinate the various services involved, including the administration of his fortnightly depot medication. A review meeting was set for three months. John participated in the development of the plan and was satisfied with the outcome. This had particular relevance given his past history of non-compliance.

Some issues for the mental health nurse
- How might non-compliance be addressed in the care plan?
- How would the needs of the carers be dealt with in the care plan?
- How can the nurse, as key worker, use the multidisciplinary team to support John?

THE SUPERVISION REGISTER

The purpose of supervision registration is to identify all people known to services who are considered to be at significant risk of committing serious violence, suicide or serious self-neglect as a result of a severe and enduring mental illness (DoH, 1994). The decision to register a person rests with the consultant psychiatrist and should be made with other members of the care team and the person's general practitioner. People identified as needing inclusion on the register are assigned to one or more of the above categories of risk. People included on the register should be informed by the consultant psychiatrist of their inclusion unless there are exceptional circumstances for not doing so, such as having an adverse effect on their mental health. The criteria for withdrawal from the register should be detailed alongside the rights of the person to access information, to request removal from the register and to request a review.

The introduction of the supervision register was an attempt to formalize multidisciplinary and multiagency risk assessment. The supervision register is aimed at people who move around between different areas and services so that new localities can be aware of the risks that they might present to themselves or others.

CASE STUDY 3.2   THE ROLE OF THE MENTAL HEALTH NURSE IN THE SUPERVISION REGISTER

John's care plan seemed to work well for the first two months and regular contact was maintained with the supporting services. However, he failed to attend the mental health centre for two successive depot injections and it was later discovered that he had also left the family home after another argument. His family had been 'too embarrassed' to inform the nurse of the dispute. The nurse also found out that John had been sacked from work for threatening a colleague again. The police were not called and no charges were brought. His threatening behaviour had never really stopped since his last period of sickness from work even though it had not been as overt as previously. This was believed to be consistent with his paranoia. The store manager had left a number of messages on his parents' answerphone but had no answer, again due to their embarrassment. Eventually the store manager contacted John's GP who in turn informed the nurse of these events. Simultaneously, the nurse had been trying to contact John after his parents informed him that he was now living with a group of friends whom they disapproved of because they were known to be regular drug users. The nurse checked the new address and found it to be an empty council flat.

The mental health team were then informed that John was held in custody in a police station in the next town. He had been arrested for assaulting and robbing a busker. It later transpired that he had been living in a squat and was now using cannabis and crack cocaine on a regular basis. He had lost two stone in weight and appeared gaunt and unkempt. He was suffering from paranoid delusions but was persuaded to go to hospital for treatment. John was quickly stabilized on antipsychotic medication and was keen to be discharged although he had no accommodation. A care programme review meeting was convened where a consensus was reached that John should be placed on the local supervision register as he was considered to be at significant risk of committing serious violence. He was discharged to a social services hostel that had 24-hour on-site staff.

By including John on the register, it was hoped that his needs would be met and that it would raise the profile of the risks associated with him. It would also enable other statutory agencies, such as social services and other health authorities, to check his risk behaviour against the register. John argued against this and felt it to be oppressive. He was concerned about being labelled as dangerous and argued that it would affect his chances of being rehoused. However, inclusion on the register went ahead despite his protestations.

Some issues for the mental health nurse

- What issues were raised for the nurse when John was missing appointments and could not be traced?
- What are the implications for the therapeutic relationship of John's inclusion on the supervision register?
- How can the nurse demonstrate that risk assessment is ongoing?

The supervision register has attracted substantial criticism. First, the legal status of the guidance came under scrutiny given the implications for the liberty of individuals and subsequent possible disclosure of confidential information (Baker, 1997; Harrison, 1994). Further criticisms highlighted the onerous requirements of the supervision register and the confusing definitional matters in mental health law (Prins, 1995). The description of 'risk' in the text accompanying the introduction has been considered too wide when compared with the description of mental illness in section 1 of the Mental Health Act (1983) (Caldicott, 1994; Hoggett, 1996).

A survey of risk registers in operation in other countries suggests, paradoxically, that the effect of the register might be to relax vigilance and control (Prins, 1995). This can be explained by the fact that placing an individual on the register can be perceived as taking adequate action and thus replaces more proactive forms of intervention (Baker, 1997).

THE MENTAL HEALTH (PATIENTS IN THE COMMUNITY) ACT 1995

The Act came into force on 1 April 1996 and made three amendments to section 25 of the Mental Health Act (1983):

1. **Leave of absence:** Extends to 12 months the period for which people detained in hospital may be given leave of absence.
2. **Absence without leave:** Extends the period during which an absconded person may be taken into custody from 28 days to six months.
3. **Supervision orders:** As with all parts of the amendment, people must be over 16 and have been compulsorily detained under the Mental Health Act (1983) and therefore be subject to section 117. Further, there must be a substantial risk of serious harm to self or others if the person does not receive aftercare and there is a strong likelihood that the person will not comply with aftercare. A named supervisor has powers to 'take and convey' and ensure that a 24-hour package of care is in place. The keyworker appointed through the CPA will usually be the supervisor and could be a nurse. This is the most significant part of the amendment and will be considered in greater detail hereafter as supervised discharge.

For some time following the implementation of the Mental Health Act (1983) mental health practice dealt with the issue of assertive follow-up in the community by using *leave of absence* available under the Act for people compulsorily detained; under section 17 home leave could be granted. Compulsory detained people were allowed home leave and recalled to the hospital before their section expired, sometimes for one night, and so were technically readmitted. They could then be discharged again, allowing them to be placed again on section 3 (treatment order) for a further six months. This practice has been referred to as 'the long leash'

Box 3.2

The scope of supervised discharge

1. Under a supervision order a person can be required to:
   - reside at a specific place;
   - attend for medical treatment;
   - attend education or training.
2. The named supervisor has a right of access to the residence of the mentally ill person, which is legally enforceable.
3. The supervisor can take and convey the person to the specified residence or for attendance for treatment, education or training and must have written authority showing they can do this.
4. The supervision order lasts initially for six months, but may be renewed for another six months and then at yearly intervals if necessary.
5. The supervision order ceases if the person is compulsorily admitted to hospital or taken into guardianship under the Mental Health Act 1983.
6. Appeals can be made to the mental health review tribunal (MHRT).

CASE STUDY 3.3 THE ROLE OF THE MENTAL HEALTH NURSE IN SUPERVISED DISCHARGE

After being included on the supervision register, John was discharged from hospital and moved into the hostel. Initially he reported that he was happy in this new environment but after a six-week period he was spending most days away from the hostel. On a couple of occasions he had stayed out overnight with a group of known drug users. He refused to discuss this with the hostel staff and insisted that he was not doing anything wrong. Whilst there was no compulsion for him to stay at the hostel, the rules required him to inform the officer in charge if he would be staying out overnight (largely to do with fire regulations and to reflect the two-way nature of the relationship). Not long after, he was absent without leave (AWOL) from Friday to Monday afternoon and missed his depot medication. Hostel staff contacted the nurse and his depot was given on the Tuesday when he returned. He was apologetic for not informing staff that he would be away and reported that he was visiting friends in 'the north'. A mental state examination revealed nothing untoward or any reason to be concerned. The nurse discussed with John the concerns of the hostel staff about spending so much time away from the hostel and his possible use of crack cocaine and cannabis. John denied using drugs and asserted his right to move about as he wished. He reluctantly agreed to weekly visits from the nurse. Hostel staff were involved in the discussions and all parties claimed they were satisfied with the outcome.

After a couple of weeks John returned late one evening in a dishevelled and disorientated state. Staff could smell alcohol on his breath but suspected that he had also been using crack cocaine again. This incident was reported to his nurse (as key worker) who visited him the following day. He was irritable and uncommunicative and said he had had too much to drink. The nurse arranged a CPA follow-up meeting for three weeks later when all the relevant parties were able to attend. In the intervening weeks John continued to use the hostel solely as a place to sleep.

At the CPA review John acknowledged this behaviour but argued that he had friends a few miles away which helped break the monotony of hostel life. After some discussion, John decided that the hostel had some responsibility for him and agreed to return by 9 pm each evening. All concerned were satisfied that John was well mentally and attributed this to his compliance with depot medication. The nurse suggested that John attend a 'back to work' programme and agreed at the meeting to initiate this with John and support him through it. A further review was agreed for three months later with the nurse to have weekly contact offering support and monitoring for his mental health.

He continued to default on the CPA plan as he continued to be AWOL and missed two further depot injections. Six weeks later he went missing and no further contact was made until the consultant psychiatrist was telephoned by the police in another city where he was detained following a serious assault on a homeless person selling magazines.

Some issues for the mental health nurse

- How could a supervised discharge provide more support than the supervision register or the initial CPA?
- What are the practical implications of *assertive follow-up* in this case?
- What contingency plans could be made in case John fails to comply with the order?

(Bean & Mounser, 1993). The effect was to produce a long-term community treatment order even though this was not in the spirit of the Act. The decisions in *Regina* v. *Hallstrom (1985)* and *Regina* v. *Gardiner (1986)* ruled that this was an unlawful use of section 17. However, the practice continues today under Scottish law although it is monitored by the Mental Welfare Commission for Scotland (Ritchie *et al.*, 1994).

Similar powers have been implemented in Victoria state in Australia and in almost every state in the USA. Studies suggest that such powers are little more than a mechanism for streamlining the admission procedures in cases of non-compliance (Dedman, 1990; McCafferty & Dooley, 1990). There is an emphasis on compulsion that erodes civil liberties and does not encourage people to engage with services. From the supervisor's point of view it is likely that these pressures will result in a reluctance by mental health workers to deal with unwilling people, as has already been seen in the USA and Australia (Dedman, 1990; Miller, 1992). Care plans need to carefully consider what contingencies can be made if the person refuses to comply with the order. Would the supervisor take the person to an outpatient clinic if they refused to go and how would they do this? Would the police become involved in such a case and how would this be of benefit to the person? Supervised discharge should only be considered when all other avenues have been explored and considered unsuitable.

The present legislation allows for people who do not comply with treatment to have their care reviewed. A number of options can be considered: a change in the services provided, a change in the requirements placed on the person, discharge from the supervision order or compulsory admission to hospital. The person is also consulted at each stage of the process by the clinical team. This consultation will elicit the views of the person and possibly encourage some form of compliance with the order. Dedman (1990) found that there are some people 'who are impressed or intimidated' by the order and whose compliance is certainly helped by it. However, 'Those cases of persuading the persuadable may represent the only situation where the order can be seen as having a useful outcome'. Additional questions arise when we consider the types of treatment that can be practically achieved in a supervisory relationship. It is conceivable that much of the focus for interventions will be one way – monitoring mental health state and ensuring compliance with depot neuroleptic medication. In this light, supervised discharge raises ethical questions about forcing people to take medication which may have unpleasant and disabling side-effects and may not be of benefit to them (Mental Health Act Commission, 1986). Further questions have been raised about the varied therapeutic benefits of such medication (MIND, 1987). However, if nothing else, this legislation requires services to consider in great detail how they are going to meet complex needs.

The main assumption underpinning supervised discharge is that it is possible to transfer controls from the hospital to the community and, indeed, that ethically it is desirable to do so (Eastman, 1994). However, this has been countered on the basis that hospital consent procedures centre around whether the person has a right to refuse to take medication. In the community, consent is about a person's right to refuse to take medication in a setting in which they are reasonably competent to operate (MIND, 1987).

CONCLUSION

Mental health nurses play a key role in the implementation of policy and legislation. They are frequently the closest professional to the service user when delivering care in both hospital and community settings. The important role mental health nurses play in hospital settings is recognized in section 5(4) of the Mental Health Act (1983). The increase in the use of this power since its introduction probably reflects the increasing demands on acute admission beds. However, it also reflects the confidence of mental health nurses in managing crises in this area.

The introduction of the CPA, in 1991, gave mental health nurses clear responsibilities as key workers for the management and treatment of mentally ill people in community settings. More recently, the introduction of the supervision register and supervised discharge has ensured that mental health nurses will feature significantly in delivering care in the community to those with the greatest need. The development of policy and legislation has shown a trend towards extending the influence of the mental health nurse in the delivery of care. While this is good for the profession, enabling it to grow and develop, mental health nurses need to be aware that with increased responsibility comes increased accountability.

REFERENCES

Ashmore, R. (1992) Factors influencing psychiatric nurses' use of section 5(4). *Nursing Times*. 88:35, 44–47.

Audit Commission (1994) *Finding a Place: A Review of Mental Health Services for Adults*. London: HMSO.

Baker, E. (1997) The introduction of supervision registers in England and Wales: a communication analysis. *Journal of Forensic Psychiatry*. 8:1, 15–35.

Bean, P. & Mounser, P. (1993) *Discharged from Mental Hospitals*. Basingstoke: Macmillan/ MIND.

Caldicott, F. (1994) Supervision registers: the College's response. *Psychiatric Bulletin*. 18, 385–386.

Cooper, S.A. & Harper, R. (1992) Section 5(2): who acts as the consultant's nominated deputy? *Psychiatric Bulletin.* 16, 759–761.

Dedman, P. (1990) Community treatment orders in Victoria, Australia. *Psychiatric Bulletin.* 14, 462–464.

Department of Health (1990) *The Care Programme Approach.* London: HMSO.

Department of Health (1993) *Factors Influencing the Implementation of the Care Programme Approach.* London: HMSO.

Department of Health (1994) *Guidance on the Discharge of Mentally Disordered People and Their Continuing Care in the Community.* London: HMSO.

Department of Health (1995) *Social Services Departments and the Care Programme Approach: An Inspection.* London: HMSO.

Department of Health (1996) *Building Bridges: A Guide to Arrangements for Inter-agency Working for the Care and Protection of Severely Mentally Ill People.* London: The Stationery Office.

Department of Health (1997a) *The Patient's Charter: Mental Health Services.* London: The Stationery Office.

Department of Health (1997b) *Statistical Bulletin: In-patients Formally Detained in Hospitals Under the Mental Health Act 1983 and Other Legislation, England: 1990–91 to 1995–96.* London: The Stationery Office.

Department of Health and the Welsh Office (1993) *Code of Practice. Mental Health Act 1983.* London: HMSO.

Eastman, N. (1994) Mental health law: civil liberties and the principle of reciprocity. *British Medical Journal.* 308, 43–45.

Harrison, K. (1994) Supervision in the community. *New Law Journal.* 144, 1017.

Hoggett, B. (1996) *Mental Health Law,* 4th edn. London: Sweet & Maxwell.

Lelliott, P. Audini, B. & Darroch, N. (1995) Resolving London's bed crisis: there might be a way, is there a will? *Psychiatric Bulletin.* 19, 273–275.

McCafferty, G. & Dooley, J. (1990) Involuntary out-patient commitment: an update. *Mental and Physical Disability Law Reporter.* 14:3, 277–287.

Mental Health Act Commission (1986) *Compulsory Treatment in the Community: A Discussion Paper.* Nottingham: MHAC.

Mental Health Act Commission (1997) *The National Visit: A One-day Visit to 309 Acute Psychiatric Wards by the Mental Health Act Commission in Collaboration with the Sainsbury Centre for Mental Health.* London: Sainsbury Centre for Mental Health.

Miller, R. (1992) Out-patient civil commitment of the mentally ill: an overview and update. *Behavioural Sciences and the Law.* 6:1, 99–118.

MIND (1987) *Compulsory Treatment in the Community.* London: MIND.

Muijen, M. (1996) Scare in the community: Britain in moral panic. In: T. Heller, J. Reynolds, R. Gomm, R. Muston & S. Pattison. (eds) *Mental Health Matters: A Reader.* London: Macmillan, pp. 143–155.

Prins, H. (1995) 'I've got a little list' (Koko: Mikado). But is it any use? Comments on the forensic aspects of 'supervision registers' for the mentally ill. *Medicine, Science and the Law.* 35, 218–224.

Regina v. Hallstrom (1985) ex Parte W. 2 ALL E.R 306.

Regina v. Gardiner (1986) ex Parte L. 2 WLR 883.

Ritchie, J., Dick, D. & Lingham, R. (1994) *The Report of the Inquiry into the Care and Treatment of Christopher Clunis.* London: HMSO.

Schneider, J. (1993) Care programming in mental health: assimilation and adaptation. *British Journal of Social Work.* 23, 383–403.

Shah, A.H. (1993) An increase in violence among psychiatric in-patients: real or apparent? *Medicine, Science and the Law.* 33:3, 227–230.

4 ORGANIZATIONAL RESPONSES TO CRISIS AND RISK: ISSUES AND IMPLICATIONS FOR MENTAL HEALTH NURSES

Mike Doyle

INTRODUCTION

Throughout history, mental health nurses have been expected to assess and manage crises and risks associated with the people they care for. Mental health service providers have also been expected to have risk assessment and management systems in place which can respond in times of crisis. Approaches to the management of risk have tended to be implicit in the practice of nurses and in the strategic direction of mental health service providers. It could be argued that crisis and risk management are nothing new to nurses or to the organizations in which they work. However, in recent times there has been a greater emphasis on the need for mental health service providers to adopt clear strategies to manage the risks facing the organization, service users, employees, visitors and members of the public. Risk management is certainly high on the current political, managerial, legal and academic agendas. It embraces a variety of concepts and pervades virtually all aspects of health care. It should aim to involve the clinical team in minimizing clinical risk and periods of crisis and therefore avoid negligence.

Mental health nurses have a key role to play in risk management generally and specifically in assessing and managing clinical risks. The characteristics of risk will be considered before looking at the reasons for the recent interest in organizational and clinical risk management in mental health services.

Occasionally, service users experience periods of acute difficulty or crisis. At these times risk of harm or loss to the service user, staff, the public and the organization may be very high. This is especially true in the era of community care where service users may be under less supervision than traditionally provided in an institution. Crisis management is synonymous with risk management in that the same principles apply. During periods of crisis the aim is to restore the service user to a balanced state and to minimize the risk of harm to the service user, members of the public, mental health staff and the organization. Therefore the management of crisis may be viewed as part of the risk management process. Models of crisis management are considered and a risk management cycle is proposed as a framework for managing risk and crisis.

The roles of nurses and the health care organizations they work within are inextricably linked when managing risk in order to minimize harm and loss. Mental health nurses need to be aware of the principles of risk management in order to avoid complaints and litigation against themselves and their organization.

Suggestions are made here which mental health nurses may find useful in minimizing risk.

CHARACTERISTICS OF RISK, RISK ASSESSMENT AND RISK MANAGEMENT

Risk means different things to different people. A typical dictionary definition may define risk as the possibility of meeting danger or harm. Definitions of risk nearly always include reference to the likelihood (possibility) of a harmful outcome (danger or harm). Risk defined in this way is sometimes referred to as *pure risk*. However, some definitions make reference to the likelihood of outcomes that may be beneficial. For example, [risk is] 'the possibility of beneficial and harmful outcomes and the likelihood of their occurrence in a stated timescale' (Alberg *et al.*, 1996). This is sometimes referred to as *speculative risk*. This definition is particularly pertinent for clinicians making decisions which involve taking risks. Risk taking is commonplace in clinical mental health services. Reaching a decision about what interventions are required to reduce or eliminate risk involves carefully weighing up the harms and benefits associated with those interventions. Most approaches to risk management initially concentrate on identifying and assessing pure risks in order to reduce or eliminate the likelihood of harmful outcomes. Risk taking arises in clinical practice when decisions are made about what measures should be implemented to reduce risks, especially when attempting to promote the independence of service users (Ryan, 1993).

Reference to risk assessment can be found in a variety of different areas. Risk assessment and management are approaches applied in the finance and insurance industry (Institute of Chartered Accountants, 1997), criminal justice system (Kemshall, 1996), health and safety management (Health & Safety Executive, 1995) and, of course, in health care services (National Health Service Executive [NHSE], 1996). If we accept the definition of pure risk, then risk assessment can be defined as the attempt to establish the level of risk, taking into account the likelihood, frequency and immediacy of harm and the severity of the possible outcomes. It is an inexact science as levels of risk are based on probabilities and not certainty. Essentially, the assessment of risk is undertaken to decide which risk management measures are required to minimize the risk of harm and increase the likelihood of benefits for the person being assessed and all those concerned (Royal College of Nursing [RCN], 1997). Once the risk has been assessed and rated then the next stage is to manage it. Risk management may be defined as the systematic, organized effort to eliminate or reduce the likelihood of misfortune, harm, damage or loss. The emphasis of this definition is on minimizing risks which result in harmful outcomes in order to maximize the benefits for all those concerned. Vital requirements of any approach to risk management are the means by which the risk of harm is reduced or eliminated. These are usually referred to as 'control measures'. Due to the connotations of the word 'control' in mental health services, a more appropriate term may be 'risk management measures' which are simply the means by which the risks are minimized.

WHY THE CURRENT INTEREST IN ORGANIZATIONAL RISK MANAGEMENT?

Although the management of risk has always been a feature of health care provision to some degree, in recent times there has been a greater emphasis on how this is actually achieved. There are many reasons for this. From an organizational perspective all mental health care providers have been subject to many changes which have made risk management crucial to the viability of their organizations.

In respect of NHS providers, in 1990 Crown Indemnity was introduced which meant that all district health authorities were vicariously liable for the actions of all their staff, including medical staff. This meant all costs following a successful clinical negligence claim would normally be met by the employing authority. Following the NHS and Community Care Act (1990), NHS trusts arrived as self-managed units. Central assistance became less likely as NHS trusts became financially independent. In turn, this meant that trusts became vicariously liable for their employees and therefore liable for all the losses arising due to insurance and legal claims. The fact that NHS bodies were liable for the negligent acts and omissions of all their employees was emphasized by the NHSE (1996) who made it clear that NHS bodies must not seek to recover costs from health care staff. The present cost of health care litigation to the NHS is estimated at £200 million per annum and is expected to rise at nearly 25% per annum over the next five years (Tingle, 1997a).

Trusts have the option of joining the Clinical Negligence Scheme for Trusts (CNST) (CNST, 1996); a pay-as-you-go mutual pooling scheme designed to assist trusts in meeting costs of clinical negligence claims. Membership of the CNST does not come cheap and some trusts may find the financial contributions prohibitive.

In April 1991 the NHS finally lost its immunity to prosecution under health and safety legislation. The effect of this is considerable as now substantial claims can be made against NHS trusts as a result of litigation following breaches of the Health and Safety at Work Act (1974). A landmark case involving Swindon and Marlborough NHS Trust (*Guardian*, 1997) confirmed the Health and Safety Executive's commitment to prosecuting trusts that do not have adequate risk management arrangements.

Trusts are now required to have elaborate complaints systems in place (Department of Health [DoH], 1995). This has made it easier for service users to make complaints which may lead to litigation and losses, especially if the complaint is not handled well.

The combined effect of these changes means that NHS trusts now face significant financial risks which could certainly impact on clinical practice standards and, in theory, could threaten the very existence of the organization. Therefore, the need for risk management strategies is clear. In 1993, in response to this, the NHSE published its document *Risk Management in the NHS* to give guidance to health care organizations on the need for and methods of introducing the management of risk in health care. The document proposes that a comprehensive risk management programme needs to be implemented to address all parts of the organization from clinical services to the management of waste. The document considered the background and principles of risk management, direct and indirect service user care risk, health and safety risk, organizational risk and methods of implementing effective risk management. The stages of managing risk consist of identifying, assessing, implementing and monitoring control measures and reviewing their efficacy. These stages are relevant for all NHS trusts: acute, community and/or mental health and health care providers in the independent sector.

THE AIM OF ORGANISATIONAL RISK MANAGEMENT

Organizations providing mental health care need to develop risk management strategies which can be implemented throughout services and departments. Ultimately, the aim of any risk management strategy should be to protect the assets of the organization. Organizations need to develop strategies aimed at creating a co-ordinated, systematic and focused approach to the management of risks in order to:

- ensure service users receive good-quality care and treatment which is safe and effective;
- ensure staff are able to work in a safe environment;
- reduce the frequency and severity of untoward incidents;
- lead to better communication and co-operation throughout the organization;
- avoid litigation and financial losses;
- introduce cost stabilization.

As clinicians, nurses' main concern will be with ensuring service users receive good-quality care and treatment which is safe and effective. If this is accomplished then the chances of meeting the other objectives will be greatly improved. This is best achieved in an environment of honesty and openness, where risks are identified quickly and dealt with in a positive and responsive way. Ideally, the response to risks should be proactive where the risk of harm is minimized by preventive measures so that crises are avoided. It is unrealistic to expect organizations to prevent all risk situations involving service users from deteriorating into crisis without the imposition of impractical and unacceptable restrictions. It is inevitable that, regardless of how well organized a mental health organization may be, some service users will experience periods of acute difficulty and crisis.

WHY THE CURRENT INTEREST IN CLINICAL RISK MANAGEMENT IN MENTAL HEALTH SERVICES?

Providers of mental health care can manage their risks in a number of ways. Risk management strategies may attempt to reduce the number of complaints and claims, try and raise clinical standards, improve health and safety practices or simply focus on saving money. Ideally, health care providers need to consider all these areas as they all impact on each other. Mental health care providers do not escape the need to develop risk management strategies. In addition to the corporate and non-clinical risks that all providers face, there is growing interest in clinical risk management in mental health services (for example, see Borum, 1996; Carson, 1996a; Monahan & Steadman, 1994, 1996; Mullen, 1997; NHS Health Advisory Service, 1994; NHSE, 1994a,b; Reed, 1997; RCP, 1996; Snowden, 1997; Steering Committee, 1996).

Mental health professionals have been expected to assess and manage risks posed by people with mental health problems for many years. In recent times there has been increasing interest in assessing and managing risks, particularly risk of self-harm and suicide, harm to others and severe self-neglect (NHSE, 1994b). There are a number of reasons for this.

Since the 1950s, successive governments have continued the policy of care in the community for people with mental health problems. This is illustrated by the fact that since the 1960s 100,000 psychiatric beds have closed in the UK (Health Committee, 1994). Assuming that the prevalence of mental health problems has at least remained the same, those who were once automatically cared for in the controlled environment of a psychiatric ward are now cared for in the community. Clearly this has raised public anxiety and the perception prevails that users of mental health services are a risk to others (Monahan, 1992; Reda, 1996).

Although care in the community is widely accepted as a desirable policy, it does seem to have reinforced public anxiety about the risks posed by mentally ill people. Public perception that users of mental health services are a greater risk to themselves and others may have been fuelled further by the number of high-profile tragedies involving people with serious mental illness. Inquiries have gained widespread media coverage with extremely negative publicity for mental health services, most notably the Clunis Inquiry (Ritchie *et al.*, 1994) and *The Falling Shadow* (Blom-Cooper *et al.*, 1995). More recent examples include the Jason Mitchell Inquiry (Blom-Cooper *et al.*, 1996), the Mursell Report (Crawford *et al.*, 1997) and the Kopernik-Steckel Inquiry (Greenwell *et al.*, 1997). The current plethora of inquiries is mainly due to the directive stated in the 'If things go wrong' section of the *Guidance on the Discharge of Mentally Disordered People and Their Continuing Care in the Community* (NHSE, 1994a). This also contained guidance on assessing risk. Each inquiry highlights specific deficits in the care and treatment provided. However, there are recurring themes in relation to:

- failure by clinicians to obtain sufficient information about a service user's history;
- poor communication between disciplines;
- poor collaboration between agencies;
- lack of clinical supervision for staff;
- lack of resources;
- failure to adequately assess and manage risk.

In 1992 the *Health of the Nation* White Paper selected mental illness as a key area for action. The aim was to reduce ill health and death caused by mental illness. To achieve this, targets were set to reduce the overall suicide rate by 15% and by 33% among severely mentally ill people by the year 2000 (DoH, 1993). Effective risk assessment and management are vital if these targets are to be achieved.

The Care Programme Approach (CPA) was introduced in 1991 to provide a framework for the care of mentally ill people outside hospital (DoH, 1990). For a fuller discussion of the CPA, the reader is referred to Chapter 3 of this volume. Operating the CPA effectively means making an assessment of risk as part of discharge planning (DoH, 1996).

Supervision registers were introduced in an attempt to prioritize care for people with serious mental illness (NHSE, 1994b). The criteria for inclusion on a supervision register are that the individual must be suffering from a serious mental illness and/or personality disorder and must pose a significant risk of self-harm, harm to others or severe self-neglect. Supervision registers can assist in targeting services for those with the most severe mental health problems, primarily on the basis of risk (Kingdon, 1996).

The Boyd Report (Steering Committee, 1996) investigated homicides and suicides committed by mentally ill people. One of the recommendations stated that employing agencies should ensure that all staff coming into direct contact with severely mentally ill persons should receive training in assessing risk. The conclusion was that clinical teams needed to strengthen risk assessment skills.

More recently, risk assessment has become even more prominent with the advent of supervised discharge legislation from 1 April 1996 (Her Majesty's Stationery Office [HMSO], 1995). The purpose of supervised discharge is to ensure that a service user who has been detained in hospital for treatment receives the aftercare services provided under section 117 of the Mental Health Act (1983). The decision as to whether a service user is subject to supervised discharge relies heavily on the level of risk to the health and safety of the service user, to the safety of other people or to the service user due to serious exploitation. Clearly risk assessment and management are central to this legislation.

The 1997 White Paper *The New NHS: Modern • Dependable* (DoH, 1997) imposed a new duty of clinical governance on NHS trusts. In brief, this requires health care providers to adopt a set framework to assure quality levels. The proposals to assure quality are very similar to the components of recognized good practice in risk management. Clinical governance requires health care providers to ensure that:

- clinical audit is in place;
- leadership skills are developed at clinical team level;
- evidence based practice is in use;
- good practice and ideas are disseminated;
- clinical risk reduction programmes are in place;

- adverse events are detected, openly investigated and lessons learned;
- lessons are learned from complaints;
- poor clinical performance is identified early;
- professional development programmes reflect principles of clinical governance;
- high-quality data are collected to monitor clinical care.

In summary, clinical risk assessment and management are high on the current clinical, managerial and legal agendas. Nurses and others working in mental health services need useful frameworks to guide their approach to risk assessment and management in order to be effective in dealing with clinical risks. As times of crisis are times of particularly high risk, then risk management frameworks should facilitate approaches to crisis prevention and management.

CRISIS MANAGEMENT

Risk management and crisis management in clinical mental health services share the same aim of reducing or eliminating the likelihood of harm to the service user and to others. It could be argued that crisis management is simply one form of risk management and part of a continuous process. Crisis management must aim to minimize the risks posed by service users experiencing periods of acute difficulty.

There are many types of crisis service in mental health care. Service users may experience crisis situations in hospital, other formal care establishments or in the community. In a hospital setting, crisis and high-risk situations are contained in a number of ways including close observation, increased staffing, administration of medication, control and restraint and psychological techniques such as anger management and de-escalation. Placement in alternative environments may be considered. Psychiatric intensive care units (PICUs) are environments which provide a higher level of nursing intervention to deal with high-risk situations. Service users who present significant risk of harm to others or property, risk of suicide and self-harming behaviour, absconding and unpredictability may benefit from intensive therapy in PICUs (Dix, 1995).

In the community, crisis services should aim to respond rapidly in order to reduce the risk of harm to the service user and others. Some services facilitate rapid admission to inpatient services with the back-up of teams working in the community while others attempt to keep service users out of hospital by providing support to people and their families in the community (Murray Parkes, 1992). A common criticism of the admission to hospital approach is that often service users have to wait until their problems have created an emergency and the risk of self-harm and/or harm to others is greatly increased. Users argue that this is expensive and does not meet their needs (Ford & Kwakwa, 1996). This view was supported by the Audit Commission (1994) report *Finding a Place*, which highlighted the increasing pressure on hospital beds and the fact that most of the mental health budget goes on the hospital acute units at the expense of community alternatives.

Therefore a vicious circle emerges which puts great pressure on beds and as a result the risk of harm is increased.

Teevan (1994) described a range of models of crisis management as alternatives to hospital admission. These include home treatment services, intensive support at home, crisis intervention service and unstaffed flats with a phone link to an acute ward. Recent research has indicated that the effectiveness of home-based approaches to the care of seriously mentally ill people has at least been equal, if not superior, to hospital-based approaches (Dean & Gadd, 1990; Marks *et al.*, 1994). Although there are clear advantages to the community model of mental health services for crisis management, working in less controlled environments away from hospital may increase risks, especially if regular contact with the service user is not maintained. Community crisis services may prevent crisis situations developing. They may also attract people to services who would otherwise be lost because of the fear of involuntary detention. Beer *et al.* (1995) describe a crisis team where the emphasis is on a proactive approach. Services are designed to encourage and maintain contact with the service user through a walk-in self-referral centre, a continuing care service and a crisis intervention service. The key to successful crisis management here is ensuring that services are accessible and able to respond rapidly when required.

Huxley & Kerfoot (1995) proposed a typology of crisis services which identified the type of help which may be provided to service users in time of crisis. This typology expanded on the work of Segal (1990) who identified three categories of help for crises: supportive, supplemental and substitutive. Huxley & Kerfoot (1995) linked this with the problem type to develop their typology of mental health crisis services (Table 4.1). The decision on which measures to use is dependent upon the problem type but will also rely on the level of risk present. The risk level should determine the response. This is reflected in the 'significant risk' category adopted in the *Guidance for Supervision Registers* (NHSE, 1994b) which aims to prioritize care for those service users falling into this category.

Table 4.1

A typology of mental health crisis services

| | Problem type | | |
Help type	Trauma	Acute illness	Long-term illness
Supportive help	Helpline Counsellor GP	Phone access Carers GP	Drop-in Care team Carers GP
Supplemental help	Groups Volunteers Outpatients	Treatment Outpatients	Case manager Key worker Volunteer
Substitutive help	Admission, if suicidal	Urgent admission	Brief admissions Foster care

(Source: Huxley & Kerfoot (1995). Reproduced with kind permission of Carfax Publishers)

Those found to be at significant risk following a risk assessment are placed on a supervision register which, in theory at least, should prioritize the care the person receives. The need to link the level of risk to the measures implemented seems to be gaining support (Monahan & Steadman, 1996). Crisis situations occur when there may be a significant risk of harm which is usually imminent. A systematic approach to risk management should therefore prove useful as a framework in which crises can be managed. Risk management progresses through the stages of identification, assessment, control/management, monitoring and review which can be illustrated as a cycle (Fig. 4.1) (Doyle, 1998; RCN, 1997).

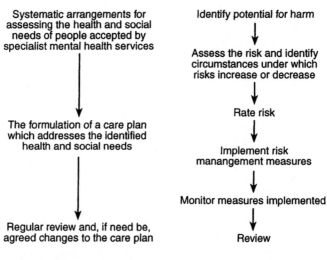

Further requirements of CPA and risk management:
• The appointment of a key worker to keep in close touch with the service user and monitor care
• Urgent review in the event of the care plan breaking down
• Collaboration with user, carer and other professionals
• Discharge from hospital only when the necessary care and support are available

Figure 4.1

Convergence of the CPA and the risk management cycle.

THE RISK MANAGEMENT CYCLE

Nearly all approaches to risk management progress through the stages of identification, assessment, control/management, monitoring and review. This is the case whether the intention is to manage the risk to service users, staff, visitors, the service or organization. The approach may be summarized as a risk management cycle (Fig. 4.1) which can easily be applied to the management of organizational and health and safety risks. Here, it is proposed as a useful framework to aid mental health nurses to assess and manage clinical risk (RCN, 1997) and therefore crisis situations. In clinical risk management, the cycle is compatible with the CPA which provides a framework for planning care for service users. Clinical risk assessment and management should be a simultaneous process to the stages of the CPA in order to manage high-risk and crisis situations effectively.

Stages of the risk management cycle

Identification of the potential for harm

The first stage in the risk management cycle is to identify if there is the potential for harm to self or others. Once this has been identified then the risk of it occurring can be assessed.

Risk assessment

The risk assessment is concerned with estimating the level of risk. This may be aided by considering the following questions.

- What is the likelihood of harm to others occurring?
- How often is it likely to occur?
- What are the possible outcomes should the harm occur?
- Who is at risk?
- How immediate is the risk?
- Over what timescale is the risk being assessed?
- Under what circumstances is the risk likely to increase/decrease?

It is unlikely that there will be definite answers to these questions. However, considering them should help to inform clinical judgement. It is very important to clarify why the risk assessment is required. Actuarial and clinical factors that may be associated with an increase or decrease in the risk of harming others should be considered. As a minimum, the assessment should obtain information related to past history, current presentation and level of support and supervision available to the service user.

Rating risk

It is unlikely that the level of risk will be measured exactly but the likelihood and outcome of the risk may be combined to produce a simple risk rating. For example:

$$\text{likelihood} \times \text{severity} = \text{risk rating}$$

Frequency and immediacy may also be included to produce the risk rating. Risk can be rated categorically: very high – high – medium – low (see, for example, Monahan & Steadman, 1996). Alternatively, the level of risk may be rated numerically if a scoring system has been employed. The risk rating should determine the risk management measures required and indicate what interventions should be implemented.

Implement risk management measures

Risk management measures are the means by which the risk of harm is minimized. They may contribute to an individual's plan of care and are not necessarily restrictive. These measures should be part of an overall plan of care produced in collaboration with the service user, where possible. In order to reduce the risk and manage crisis effectively, the response to the risk needs to be considered taking into account different levels of intervention.

Roberts & Holly (1996) suggested four levels of management response necessary for minimizing risk: primary, secondary, tertiary and externally imposed. Primary measures are proactive and aim to prevent harm occurring and may include early warning systems and pre-emptive contact between key worker and service user. Secondary measures are taken during and immediately after an adverse incident and may include development of a crisis contingency plan, standby arrangements to ensure an urgent response by mental health professionals, more intensive care and possibly admission to hospital. Tertiary measures are taken to reduce the risks which arise as a consequence of any adverse incident. Change of residence or more intensive contact with service user and family may be appropriate at this stage. Care plans will usually include a combination of these measures. External legislation and guidelines may be imposed to improve risk management practices. In these circumstances, organizations and the clinicians they employ need to be aware of their existence and apply them accordingly. In clinical services, examples of these include section 117 of the Mental Health Act (1983), the CPA, supervision registers, supervised discharge and restriction orders as applied under section 41 of the Mental Health Act (1983). The more proactive a service is in identifying, assessing and managing risk, the better prepared it should be to integrate external imposed legislation and guidelines.

Before implementing risk management measures, clinicians need to carefully weigh up the harms and benefits associated with the measures and also the harms and benefits of inaction (Carson, 1990). This is very important for the service user. Also careful consideration and documentation of the harms and benefits of a decision will improve the defence of the clinician if something goes wrong. Risk decisions need to be made in a manner which can be readily justified (Carson, 1996b). A date should be agreed to review the measures implemented, usually as part of the care planning review process.

Monitoring of risk management measures

Risk management measures need to be monitored to ensure that they are being implemented as planned and in order to keep up to date on progress between reviews.

Review

The review should be concerned with evaluating whether the measures implemented have eliminated or reduced the risks. This will involve a reassessment of risk and the cycle should continue through the rating, implementation and monitoring stages, therefore continuing the risk management cycle.

REDUCING COMPLAINTS, LITIGATION AND FINANCIAL LOSSES

Mental health nurses play a key role in providing care and treatment but they often have to work in under-resourced teams with an ever-increasing number of pressures. Complaints about the NHS rose by 25% in 1994 (Health Service Commissioner, 1994). The combination of increasing workload and the rising number of complaints means that nurses are now at greater risk of being the target of complaints and possible litigation.

It is inevitable that mistakes and errors will occur in the provision of mental health services. It is the responsibility of management and staff to ensure that when a failure does occur, steps are taken for it to be resolved with the minimum harm or loss. The principal aim of risk management is to ensure service users receive good-quality care and treatment which is safe and effective. In order to achieve this, service users need to be protected from failures in health care delivery. Obviously, it is much more desirable to have proactive primary risk management measures in place to minimize the risk of harm.

Complaints and litigation against individuals and/or the organization may occur for many different reasons. Service users and others will have views and opinions about the care they receive. Organizations need to encourage service users to express their views and opinions as this can assist organizations to identify both positive and negative aspects of the service provided. In turn, this will lead to action being taken to improve services where there are failings. A well-handled complaint can reduce the risk of litigation.

NHS trusts and other mental health care providers can take proactive measures to reduce the risk of complaints and litigation. Van Liew (1997) recommends that NHS trusts need to put systems in place which identify new and emerging risks through efficient incident reporting systems as well as developing and implementing comprehensive risk management programmes. The main stages of the programme suggested are similar to those proposed in Figure 4.2.

Many mental health care organizations adopt risk management strategies. There is also a need to clarify how mental health workers can ensure good risk management practices which can contribute to organizational risk management strategies and protect the individual clinician, while ensuring service users receive the best standard of care available.

IMPLICATIONS FOR MENTAL HEALTH NURSES

As nurses are at the forefront in providing care and treatment, they need to ensure service users receive good-quality care and treatment which is safe and effective. If this is achieved then the frequency and severity of adverse incidents will be reduced and therefore complaints, litigation and financial losses should be avoided. Mental health nurses may be covered by the principles of vicarious liability where the employers are liable for the actions of all their employees. However, this does not exclude nurses from contributing to good risk management practices. There are many ways in which nurses can ensure good risk management practice. Quality

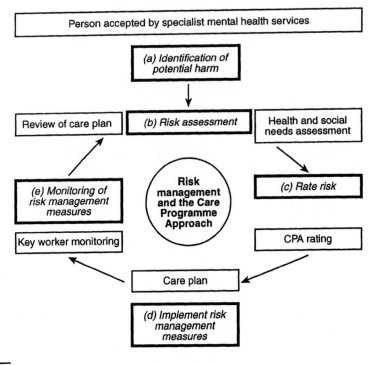

Figure 4.2

Relationship between the stages of the risk management cycle and the stages of the Care Programme Approach.

care and treatment is synonymous with good risk management practice. Organizational risk management practices are usually complementary to programmes of quality assurance, quality improvement and clinical audit (Moss, 1995).

There are numerous measures mental health nurses can take to protect themselves and the organizations they work for which in turn should result in a better quality service for the service user (Table 4.2).

CONCLUSION

Interest in risk management in mental health services continues to grow as organizations and their employees are becoming increasingly aware of the need to clarify how they identify, assess and manage risk. The characteristics of risk are open to debate. Risk assessment is an inexact science. The initial aim of risk assessment is to estimate the level of risk using all the information available while the overall aim is to minimize the risk of harm and loss while ensuring maximum benefits for all concerned. Clinical risk management in mental health services continues to attract attention as high-profile tragedies involving mentally ill people are publicized as evidence of failures in community care. Subsequent legislation

Table 4.2

Measures nurses can take to minimize risk

Measures	Rationale
Using a risk management framework	It is important for mental health nurses to adopt a framework for risk management which clearly demonstrates how the nurse identifies, assesses and manages risk. This is especially true in clinical risk management where risk taking is fundamental to the principles of rehabilitation.
Clinical supervision	Clinical supervision is intended to encourage nurses to reflect on quality control aspects of their practice. In theory at least, this should improve services, maintain standards in a rapidly evolving environment, make practice more evidence based, target resources and reduce risk through reflection and planned action.
Professional development	Mental health nurses need to continually develop their knowledge and skills in rapidly changing health care environments. This should ensure that care is delivered in a safe and effective way which is in accordance with a practice accepted as proper by their peers, thereby reducing the risk of being found negligent.
Clinical guidelines and protocols	Clinical guidelines aim to provide an evidence base for the provision of care and are being increasingly seen as clinical effectiveness tools. The development of clinical guidelines should involve all disciplines involved in the service user's care. Closely linked to clinical practice guidelines are multidisciplinary clinical protocols and care pathways which provide frameworks to improve the quality of care and therefore reduce the risk of harm or loss. Potential benefits include: • the promotion of collaborative practice amongst health care professionals; • enhancing multidisciplinary understanding of each other's roles and contributions; • promoting consistency in clinical practice; • building best practice; • clarifying processes and outcomes of care; • reducing duplication; • managing risk; • demystifying health care and empowering service users.
Good communication and documentation	It is vital that all stages of assessment and decision-making processes are clearly recorded in the service user's notes. Information should be made available to other clinicians and agencies involved in the care and treatment of the service user, provided this is in accordance with the UKCC Code of Confidentiality and/or similar local guidelines. Comprehensive, objective, consistent and accurate communication and documentation of care contribute to minimizing risk.
Involving service users (or advocates) in their care and treatment	This can help develop trust and build therapeutic relationships. Greater involvement by service users in assessment (including risk assessments), planning and implementing care should be actively encouraged by nurses and become part of routine clinical practice.
Reporting and recording of incidents and concerns	It is vital that incidents and concerns are reported at an early stage in order to avoid something more serious occurring. Also, keeping a record of all adverse incidents will allow analysis of the data so that trends may be identified.

(Compiled from the following references: BMA, 1996; Butterworth & Faugier, 1992; Campbell & Lindow, 1997; Darley, 1996; Nicholson, 1997; RCN, 1997; RCP, 1996, 1997; Tingle, 1997b; United Kingdom Central Council, 1996; Wilson, 1995)

and guidelines have focused the attention of clinicians and managers alike on the need for good clinical risk management practices. The question of how services respond to service users in crisis has become especially relevant in an era of community care where an inquiry culture prevails.

Crisis management is synonymous with risk management and may be applied using a risk management cycle. There are strategies that health care organizations can employ to minimize the risk of harm and loss which should also contribute to continuing quality improvement. Mental health nurses can also adopt measures to reduce the risks to service users, the public, themselves and the organizations in which they work.

REFERENCES

Alberg, C., Hatfield, B. & Huxley, P. (1996) *Learning Materials on Mental Health Risk Assessment*. Manchester: Manchester University and Department of Health.

Audit Commission (1994) *Finding a Place: A Review of Mental Health Services for Adults*. London: HMSO.

Beer, D., Cope, S., Smith, J. & Smith, R. (1995) The crisis team as part of comprehensive local services. *Psychiatric Bulletin*. 19, 616–619.

Blom-Cooper, L., Hally, H. & Murphy, E. (1995) *The Falling Shadow: One Patient's Mental Health Care 1978–1993*. London: Duckworth.

Blom-Cooper, L., Grounds, A., Guinan, P., Parker, A. & Taylor, M. (1996) *The Case of Jason Mitchell: Independent Panel of Inquiry*. London: Duckworth.

Borum, R. (1996) Improving the clinical practice of violence risk assessment. *American Psychologist*. 51:9, 945–956.

British Medical Association (1996) *Risk Management in the NHS*. Health Policy and Economic Research Unit. London: BMA.

Butterworth, T. & Faugier, J. (1992) *Clinical Supervision and Mentorship in Nursing*. London: Chapman & Hall.

Campbell, P. & Lindow, V. (1997) *Changing Practice: Mental Health Nursing and User Empowerment – RCN Learning Materials on Mental Health*. London: RCN/MIND.

Carson, D. (ed) (1990) *Risk Taking in Mental Disorder: Analyses, Policies and Practical Strategies*. Southampton: SLE Publications.

Carson, D. (1996a) Developing models of risk to aid co-operation between law and psychiatry. *Criminal Behaviour and Mental Health*. 6, 6–10.

Carson, D. (1996b) Risking legal repercussions. In: H. Kemshall & J. Pritchard (eds) *Good Practice in Risk Assessment and Risk Management*, Volume 1. London: Jessica Kingsley Publishers, pp. 3–12.

Clinical Negligence Scheme for Trusts (1996) *Risk Management Standards and Procedures: Manual of Guidance*. Bristol: CNST.

Crawford, L., Ferris, R. & Hayward, P. (1997) *Report into the Care and Treatment of Martin Mursell*. London: Camden and Islington Health Authority.

Darley, M. (1996) *Can Clinical Supervision Improve Risk Management?* Health Care Risk Report. London: Eclipse Group, pp. 20–21.

Dean, C. & Gadd, E.M. (1990) Home treatment for acute psychiatric illness. *British Medical Journal*. 301, 1021–1023.

Department of Health (1990) *The Care Programme Approach for People with a Mental Illness Referred to the Specialist Psychiatric Services*. London: HMSO.

Department of Health (1993) *The Health of the Nation: Key Area Handbook – Mental Illness*. London: HMSO.

Department of Health (1995) *Acting on Complaints: Revised Policy and Proposals for the New NHS Complaints Procedure in England*. London: HMSO.

Department of Health (1996) *Building Bridges: A Guide to Arrangements for Interagency Working for the Care and Protection of Severely Mentally Ill People*. London: The Stationery Office.

Department of Health (1997) *The New NHS: Modern • Dependable*. London: HMSO.

Dix, R. (1995) A nurse led psychiatric intensive care unit. *Psychiatric Bulletin*. 19, 285–287.

Doyle, M. (1998) Clinical risk assessment for mental health nurses. *Nursing Times*. 94:17, 47–49.

Ford, R. & Kwakwa, J. (1996) Rapid reaction, speedy recovery. *Health Service Journal*. 18 April, 30–31.

Greenwell, J., Procter, A. & Jones, A. (1997) *Report of the Inquiry into the Treatment and Care of Gilbert Kopernik-Steckel*. Croydon Health Authority.

Guardian (1997) Hospital trust fined £4,000 in landmark case. 21 August.

Health and Safety Executive (1995) *Five Steps to Risk Assessment*. London: HSE.

Health Committee (1994) *Better Off in the Community: The Care of People who are Seriously Mentally Ill* (First Report: Vol. 1, together with the proceedings of the committee). London: HMSO.

Health Service Commissioner (1994) *Annual Report for 1993–94*. London: HMSO.

Her Majesty's Stationery Office (1995) *Mental Health (Patients in the Community) Act*. London: HMSO.

Huxley, P. & Kerfoot, M. (1995) Letter from Manchester: a typology of crisis services for mental health. *Journal of Mental Health*. 4, 431–435.

Institute of Chartered Accountants (1997) *Business Risk Management*. London: ICAEW.

Kemshall, H. (1996) *Reviewing Risk: A Review of the Assessment and Management of Risk and Dangerousness: Implications for Policy and Practice in the Probation Service*. London: Home Office.

Kingdon, D. (1996) Supervision registers: caring or controlling? *British Journal of Hospital Medicine*. 56:9, 470–472.

Marks, I.M., Connolly, J., Muijen, M., Audini. B., McNamee, G. & Lawrence, R.E. (1994) Home-based versus hospital-based care for people with serious mental illness. *British Journal of Psychiatry*. 165, 179–194.

Monahan, J. (1992) Mental disorder and violent behaviour: perceptions and evidence. *American Psychologist*. 47:4, 511–521.

Monahan, J. & Steadman, H.J. (eds) (1994) *Violence and Mental Disorder: Developments in Risk Assessment*. Chicago: University of Chicago Press.

Monahan, J. & Steadman, H. (1996) Violent storms and violent people: how meteorology can inform risk communication in mental health law. *American Psychologist*. 51:9, 931–938.

Moss, F. (1995) Risk management and quality of care. *Quality in Health Care*. 4, 102–107.

Mullen, P. (1997) Assessing risk of interpersonal violence in the mentally ill. *Advances in Psychiatric Treatment*. 3, 163–173.

Murray Parkes, C. (1992) Perception of a crisis service by referrers and clients. *Psychiatric Bulletin*. 16, 751–753

National Health Service Executive (1993) *Risk Management in the NHS*. London: NHSE.

National Health Service Executive (1994a) *Guidance on the Discharge of Mentally Disordered People and their Continuing Care in the Community.* London: NHSE.

National Health Service Executive (1994b) *Introduction of Supervision Registers for Mentally Ill People from 1 April 1994.* London: NHSE.

National Health Service Executive (1996) *NHS Indemnity: Arrangements for Clinical Negligence Claims in the NHS.* London: NHSE.

NHS Health Advisory Service (1994) *Suicide Prevention: Mental Health Services – The Challenge Confronted.* London: HMSO.

Nicholson, J. (1997) *Care Pathways: A Tool for Improving Quality and Managing Risk.* Health Care Risk Report. London: Eclipse Group, pp. 16–17.

Reda, S. (1996) Public perceptions of former psychiatric patients in England. *Psychiatric Services.* 47:11, 1253–1255.

Reed, J. (1997) Risk assessment and clinical risk management: the lessons from recent inquiries. *British Journal of Psychiatry.* 170 (supplement 32), 4–7.

Ritchie, J.H., Dick, D. & Lingham, R. (1994) *The Report of the Inquiry into the Care and Treatment of Christopher Clunis.* London: HMSO.

Roberts, G. & Holly, J. (1996) *Risk Management in Healthcare.* London: Witherby.

Royal College of Nursing (1997) *Risk Assessment: Guidance for Mental Health Nurses: Assessing and Managing the Risk of Harm to Others from People with Mental Health Problems* (draft paper). London: RCN.

Royal College of Psychiatrists (1996) *Assessment and Clinical Management of Risk of Harm to Other People.* London: RCP.

Royal College of Psychiatrists (1997) *The Management of Violence in Clinical Settings: An Evidence Based Guideline* (draft review copy). London: RCP.

Ryan, T. (1993) Therapeutic risks in mental health nursing. *Nursing Standard.* 7: 24, 29–31.

Segal, S.P. (1990) Emergency care for the acute and severely mentally ill. In: I.M. Marks & R.A. Scott (eds) *Mental Health Care Delivery: Innovations, Impediments and Implementation.* Cambridge: Cambridge University Press, pp. 104–110.

Snowden, P. (1997) Practical aspects of clinical risk assessment and management. *British Journal of Psychiatry.* 170 (supplement 32), 32–34.

Steering Committee of the Confidential Inquiry into Homicides and Suicides by Mentally Ill People. (1996) *Report of the Confidential Inquiry into Homicides and Suicides by Mentally Ill People.* London: Royal College of Psychiatrists.

Teevan, S. (1994) *Crisis Services* (fact sheet). London: MIND Information Unit.

Tingle, J. (1997a) Healthcare litigation: working towards a culture change. *British Journal of Nursing.* 6:1, 56–57.

Tingle, J. (1997b) Clinical guidelines: legal and clinical risk management issues. *British Journal of Nursing.* 6:11, 639–640.

United Kingdom Central Council (1996) *Guidelines for Professional Practice.* London: UKCC.

Van Liew, D. (1997) Clinical risk management within the NHS. *Nursing Times Research.* 2:2, 88–96.

Wilson, J. (1995) Clinical risk modification. *British Journal of Nursing.* 4:11, 667.

PART TWO

CLINICAL NURSING PRACTICE FOR CRISIS AND RISK MANAGEMENT

5 CRISIS AND RISKS ASSOCIATED WITH SCHIZOPHRENIA

Siobhan Sharkey

INTRODUCTION

Risks for people with a diagnosis of schizophrenia are many and varied. Awareness of these risks is crucial in understanding the very personal and often chaotic experience of disrupted, delusional and hallucinatory thinking in addition to other features of schizophrenia.

As with other mental illnesses, not all risks associated with schizophrenia are crisis events. Nevertheless, some of the most acutely distressed people that nurses will work with are those who are actively experiencing psychotic symptoms. Mental health nurses need to be able to identify the risks associated with schizophrenia, which of them create the potential for a crisis and how they can help people to manage them. In addition, mental health nurses work with people with serious and enduring psychotic experiences over long time frames so they need the skills to support service users and their families through the risks associated with long-term illness. Service users with schizophrenia can experience a range of crises and can be 'at risk' as a result both of their mental illness and because of social, economic and environmental contexts (for a review, see Ryan, 1996). This chapter considers both the crises associated with schizophrenia and the longer term risks.

The detrimental effects of having a serious and enduring illness to both the service users and their carers are well known (Provencher *et al.*, 1997). Early perspectives on psychotic illnesses, and in particular those grouped as schizophrenia (World Health Organisation [WHO], 1992), emphasized the *carer* aspects of the illness and placed a great emphasis on the reduction of symptoms, often to the added detriment of the service user.

However, an important starting point for risk management in relation to schizophrenia (as argued throughout this book) is an understanding of the very individual nature of risks. Such risks are a product not only of the person's mental state or psychological condition but also historical, social, and environmental factors experienced by the service user. Attempts to understand the nature of schizophrenia and similar psychotic illnesses (whether exclusively via a symptom model or combined assessment of a person's lived experiences) are ongoing and mental health nurses need to be knowledgeable about both the range of potential causes and resultant experiences. A recent review of schizophrenia examined research in three areas: the aetiology, epidemiology and neuropsychology of schizophrenia (Gournay, 1996). However, this view has been criticized as being premature given the current research base (Dawson, 1997). Other texts discuss schizophrenia variously in terms of aetiology such as genetics, obstetric complications and life events, epidemiology, psychosocial factors, culture and age of onset (Hirsch & Weinberger, 1995; Thomas *et al.*, 1997).

The wide range of experiences associated with schizophrenia or psychosis have been grouped by the medical profession to reflect clusters of symptoms and longevity of experience. These are accessible in the *International Classification of Diseases (ICD-10)*, used mainly in Britain and Europe, and the *Diagnostic and Statistical Manual of Mental Disorders* used in America (American Psychiatric Association [APA], 1987; Hirsch & Weinberger, 1995; WHO, 1992). Categories such as schizophrenia, schizotypal disorder, persistent delusional disorder, acute and transient psychotic disorders, among others (WHO, 1992), may provide ready classifications for research purposes but reflect little of the lived experience of the service user. In terms of identifying potential risks, it is likely to be more useful to know that a service user with an enduring psychosis has limited communication rather than that they have *catatonic schizophrenia* or that they appear overzealous or gregarious in their behaviour rather than that they have *hebephrenic schizophrenia*. Boxes 5.1 and 5.2 summarize the main groupings and aetiology of schizophrenia.

Focusing on a *disease* for treatment purposes may miss the person's cluster of symptoms or experiences, which do not always follow a predictable path. Professionals may be able to trace early signs, first-episode risks and crisis events, enabling them to profile the recurring or enduring symptoms and risky events of personal experience. However, it is important that a person's prognosis is not dependent on the disease model alone. Moving beyond the disease model allows assessment to move into other aspects of an individual's life such as housing, support, employment and occupation as well as coping strategies, confidence and insight. While assessment of mental state gives important information in determining potential risks associated with particular symptoms, the assessment of psychological condition and social situation, and their impact on risks, is also crucial.

This view reflects guidance on good risk management, that is, risk assessment, risk reduction and risk-taking activities, where the use of clinical/practitioner

---

Box 5.1

Descriptive psychopathology of schizophrenia (traditional groupings)

- **Positive symptoms:** hallucinations and other abnormal experiences, delusions and catatonia.
- **Negative symptoms:** impaired attention, intelligence, memory, perception and will.
- **Psychopathological groupings:** thought disorder and disturbances of emotions.

(Based on Hirsch & Weinberger, 1995)

Box 5.2

Aetiology of schizophrenia

- **Genetic:** Studies indicate a genetic liability of 63–85% but schizophrenia is seen as a heterogeneous group of disorders.

- **Perinatal complications:** Research to date suggests that low birth weights are associated with prevalence of schizophrenia but more research is needed in this area.

- **Winter births:** People born during winter months are approximately 10% more likely to experience schizophrenia. This may be due to exposure of the mother to viral infections or epidemic strains of the flu.

- **Physiology:** Analysis of brain metabolism and CT scans have facilitated examination of brain structure. Controlled studies employing these techniques have shown abnormalities in a range of brain areas.

(Compiled from Carpenter & Buchanan, 1995; Gournay, 1996; Hirsch & Weinberger, 1995; McNeil *et al.*, 1993; Provencher *et al.*, 1997; Takei *et al.*, 1994; Thomas *et al.*, 1997)

---

interviews and actuarial data should underpin the decision-making process around high, immediate and ongoing risks (Carson, 1996; Department of Health [DoH], 1995; Ryan, 1996).

Key issues for mental health nurses managing crisis or high risk are concerned with trying to balance the risks to and from the service user. What are the positive and negative outcomes of intervention or non-intervention for the individual and what is their likelihood?

A number of serious risks and crisis events are associated with schizophrenia. These can be related to first-episode crisis and to ongoing risks which accompany an enduring psychotic illness.

FIRST-EPISODE CRISIS

An individual beginning to experience psychotic thinking and living within a very close and often conflicting family situation may eventually reach crisis point. Early psychotic experiences are particularly difficult times for the person and their family. New services and therapeutic interventions are being targeted at this group of (often) young people to try and provide a buffer effect to crisis.

However, one difficulty with first-episode or early psychosis work is the anomalous and fluctuating experiences and formation of delusional thinking which can make relationship building very difficult initially. Clear guidelines and good support for staff are essential. Many new services aim to use public health information, education assessments and psychotherapeutic techniques to intervene with those at risk through working with primary health care teams and liaising with schools (together with the general public). Research into the efficacy of this is at an early stage with questions around preventive capabilities or impact of therapies yet to be answered (Birchwood *et al.*, 1997; McGorry *et al.*, 1996).

Family confusion and increasing withdrawal or antagonism may eventually be brought to the attention of a GP or a crisis linked to a violent or self-harm attempt may precipitate hospital admission via an accident and emergency department. Research has shown that violence is frequent on psychiatric wards and while it may be imperative that an individual is admitted to hospital for safety reasons following a crisis, this may portray a controlling and hopeless message to them (Whittington, 1994). Sensitivity and safety are important aspects of nursing care for this group of service users (as with others). In addition, admission to hospital itself may heighten feelings of anxiety and persecution for people who may already feel under threat (Lipsedge, 1995).

SCHIZOPHRENIA AND VIOLENCE

Epidemiological studies have shown that people with a diagnosis of schizophrenia are more likely to have been violent than individuals without a mental illness, albeit marginally. One particular study suggested that people with schizophrenia accounted for only 3% of total violence (Swanson *et al.*, 1990). However, studies have also questioned this view. Wessely (1997) cites a number of studies which suggest that offending and violence among mentally ill people are related to their relatively higher rates of poverty and poorer family history. In addition, the existence of previous offending history before the onset of the mental illness has also been identified as a factor for subsequent offending or violence. Taylor (1995) has focused on links between schizophrenia and homicides (as the 'most serious and finite of crimes') and cautions against over interpretation of figures and suggests that 'Only a tiny minority of unlawful homicides are committed by people with schizophrenia' (Taylor, 1995, p.168). From a different perspective, Taylor & Gunn (1984) undertook a prison focused study in Brixton and found that 6% had schizophrenia and that nearly 9% of those on remand had some kind of psychotic symptoms. The evidence is not clearcut but it is obvious that belief in a strong link between mental illness and violence is extremely misguided (Monahan & Steadman, 1983).

Those experiencing active psychotic symptoms, especially delusional thinking, are thought to be particularly at risk, while other studies suggest that persecutory delusional thinking may be particularly linked with violence or delusions of control by others, whereas hallucinations are rarely acted upon (Gottleib *et al.*, 1987; Link *et al.*, 1992; Monahan & Steadman, 1994; Taylor, 1985). However, links between mental illness and violence are small compared with other groups in society (Swanson *et al.*, 1990). Key factors for violence appear to be male gender, low socioeconomic status, youth and substance misuse which highlight how minor, by comparison, the contribution of a mental illness may be (Monahan, 1992).

It may not solely be illness or delusional thinking that will dictate the immediacy of risk of violence to others. Lack of information about an individual may also increase the risk of violence occurring. A history of violence is also an indicator for future violent behaviour (Woodley *et al.*, 1995). Furthermore, the family situation and relationships can influence the likelihood of violence (as with the general population) (Gelles, 1987). People with schizophrenia may have difficulty in forming long-lasting relationships and may have a tendency toward isolation, resulting in an increased dependency on close family members. In these circumstances, conflicts within the family, coupled with increasing delusional and persecutory thinking, can provide the trigger which may lead to violent acts. It has been known for some time that random acts of violence against strangers are rare. People with schizophrenia are most likely to assault those they live with or the mental health professionals who work with them, particularly nurses (Ryan, 1996).

ASSESSING RISK OF VIOLENCE

Whether in hospital or as part of a community mental health team, it is important that nurses can assess risk of violence in order to avoid the crisis associated with such acts.

If there is an indication of previous violent behaviour and if the service user is receptive, continuing to ask for details will shed light on whether the person is considering violence and the level of any intent or planning which may be present. In addition, the nurse will be able to gain information about the link between any delusional or persecutory thinking and the continued consideration of violence.

The nurse may also be able to determine the coping ability of the service user by asking what they see as the biggest stressors in their lives and how they cope with them. This may provide information on patterns of perceived stressors or any recurring violent responses and identify similarities between people, places and methods and whether alcohol or drug use occurs in these scenarios. Such information is not going to ensure the prevention of violence in every case but will allow the formation of a management plan to cope with possible violence in the future (Monahan, 1988).

People experiencing active hallucinations or delusional thinking may not be able to answer questions for any prolonged period of time and the nurse needs to be aware of this, along with their own impact on the service user's thinking. Clarity of speech, continual checking about the service user's understanding and observation of body language will provide clues to any increase in tension. The nurse should be prepared to carefully wind down an interview session until later to avoid an escalation of anxiety or the likelihood that the service user may incorporate the nurse into their delusional thinking.

Planning with the service user to reduce the likelihood of violent behaviours should include information on:

- difficult coping areas and trigger situations;
- the service user's rationale for why they become violent;
- times of increased anxiety and whether this is linked to delusional thinking or hallucinations;

Box 5.3

Areas to investigate in assessing risk of violence

- **Risk factors:** Higher risk has been associated with youth, male gender, unemployed status, poor housing, low educational achievement, serious mental illness (particularly paranoid psychosis) and alcohol or drug misuse.
- **History:** One of the best predictors of future violence is past violence. Questions should be asked about issues such as the recency, frequency, severity and triggers of anay previous violence.
- **Ideation:** Thoughts and feeling about violence and plans to carry out violent acts should be examined. Does the person have the means to carry out an act of violence?
- **Intention:** Is the person saying they will harm a specific person? This is not always declared even though the person may be thinking of it.
- **Communication:** Nurses can use their empathic skills to sensitively ask questions regarding the above. The particular relationship the nurse has with the person will dictate the timing and pace of quesions. Do not pursue questioning if the person becomes agitated. Avoid a pushy technique. Some useful initial questions can include:

  Have you ever used force against someone?
  How close have you been to using violence?
  Have you ever thought about using violence?
  Do you feel threatened?
  Have you ever been arrested?
  Do you ever become more aggressive when you've been drinking?
  Have you ever used a weapon against someone?

(Based on McNeil *et al.*, 1993; Swanson *et al.*, 1990; Thomas *et al.*, 1997)

- identification of positive coping strategies employed by the service user to prevent violence occurring;
- drug and/or alcohol use;
- problem settings.

It may be necessary to work over a period of time with the service user to identify positive areas and reduce the risk of violence.

CRISIS INVOLVING VIOLENCE

Warning signs can provide clues to increasing tension and may indicate imminent crisis events involving violent actions. The nurse should be familiar with these

---

Box 5.4

Self-awareness during crisis associated with violent acts

- Know where your colleagues are and ensure that they know where you are.
- Know the layout of the environment and where exits are.
- Do not invade personal space and leave room for movement.
- Be aware of the potential dangers of clothing causing injury, such as scarves and earrings.
- Ensure good communication between staff about service users. If working alone, agree a check-in time with colleagues.
- Think about how you visit beforehand and avoid being alone on the first visit to someone you do not know.
- Plan your route in advance and where to park safely. Be streetwise about your visits and check the type of area with colleagues before you leave.
- Think of the best time of day to travel and try to avoid being a woman alone.
- Use a mobile phone or pager, but do not rely on it as it can slow you down or be used as a weapon against you.
- If necessary, use other agencies such as the police or social services.

---

signs so that they can adjust their own behaviour and communication to reduce tension.

A nurse may encounter violent incidents in hospital areas or may be part of a team or provide crisis cover within a community mental health team. Self-awareness and keen observation are essential in the prevention of violence. In addition, good leadership, staff support and training can improve team management of violent events. Boxes 5.4 and 5.5 summarise key points in the management of crisis associated with violent acts.

Not all the signs in Box 5.5 are likely to occur together and some may also be due to physical or neurological problems. The nurse needs to be careful to make distinctions between signs of aggression and possible physical problems. It is worth noting that these signs may also be precipitated by an individual actively experiencing hallucinations where increasing tension or aggression may be directed towards the perceived source of threat (the nurse, family members or other service users/staff).

Should a violent incident occur the immediate aims are to defuse the situation and ensure safety for all concerned. Subsequent actions should aim at support (for the service user and staff), understanding and developing new coping strategies and restoration and maintenance of the service user's esteem and positive outlook.

During an incident the nurse needs to observe verbal and non-verbal

---

Box 5.5

Signs of increasing tension and agitation

Physical
- Little or no eye contact
- Clenching and unclenching of fists
- Jerky body movements
- Continual face movements
- Rapid eye movements/dilated pupils
- Pacing up and down
- Clenching or tightening of jaw
- Increased breathing and rapid pulse

Communication
- Increased volume or pitch of voice
- Pressure of speech (rapid or disjointed)
- Swearing or abusive language
- Hostile or angry comments
- Irritable responses
- Monosyllabic responses

(Based on Alberg *et al.*, 1996; Lipsedge, 1995)

---

communications regarding the way a service user is interpreting what is being said. In some instances it may be more appropriate and safer for the nurse to withdraw and encourage others to do likewise. If the service user is increasingly agitated or distressed the use of additional medication could be considered and offered. However, the nurse must use this option with care (see Chapter 12). Awareness of the effects of antipsychotic drugs on the service user's feelings of frustration, together with their views on taking medication, is important. It is also crucial to tailor an individual response even during times of increasing tension. This is particularly true for someone who is hallucinating as they may be confused and distracted.

Strategies for physical restraint should be agreed in advance for clinical areas, carried out by more than one trained person wherever possible and should be shortlived. Intervention should be followed by support for both staff and service users. There are numerous works on violence and aggressive behaviours to which the reader is referred for greater detail (Alberg *et al.*, 1996; Monahan & Steadman, 1994; Stuart & Sundeen, 1995; Thomas *et al.*, 1997).

Box 5.6

Communication when managing violent incidents

Verbal
- Tell the service user who you are and why you are there.
- Remind the service user where they are and the reasons why.
- Show a caring and supportive role by using a preferred name.
- Say you want to help.
- Use a clear and calming voice, keeping sentences simple, short and clear.
- Stay calm and be alert for colleagues and others in the area.
- Call for a colleague if alone.
- Avoid a patronizing manner.

Non-verbal
- Adopt a non-threatening posture.
- Relax shoulders.
- Keep arms down and hands open and outwards.
- Do not stand directly in front of the person but try to keep sideways to them.
- Do not smile or grimace overtly when someone is delusional or hallucinating as this can be misinterpreted.
- Avoid potentially threatening gestures such as waving arms around, pointing, crossed arms and hands on hips.
- Try and keep all parties in an open space.
- Try not to mirror any of the service user's negative body language.
- Assess the environment and layout.

(Adapted from Alberg *et al.*, 1996; Thomas *et al.*, 1997)

RISKS OF HARM TO SELF

People with schizophrenia may also be at high and immediate risk of harming themselves. They are particularly at risk when actively delusional, hallucinating or concurrently depressed. People who suffer schizophrenia have a 10% lifetime risk of suicide (Hogman & Meier, 1995) and account for one in three hospital suicides. Depressive episodes may also be experienced, where ongoing and debilitating symptoms can increase suicide risk (Morgan & Owen, 1990). Indicators for suicide attempts and self-harm are discussed in Chapter 7. The

---

Box 5.7

Managing risk of self-harm

Crises in community settings
- Make frequent contact (home/day centres/outpatients).
- Make rapid follow-up for failed contacts (establish an agreed team plan with clear roles and responsibilities).
- Monitor medication and use optimum dose to lift mood with minimal side effects to avoid overdose.
- Build a therapeutic relationship.

Crises in hospital settings
- Provide constant supervision through close observation.
- Provide clear notes and communication.
- Clarify responsibilities within the team.
- Monitor medication and use optimum dose to lift mood with minimal side-effects to avoid overdose.
- Use power of detention (e.g. section 5(4) of the 1983 Mental Health Act) if necessary at times of crisis.
- Build a therapeutic relationship.

Long-term management of risk
- Work to an agreed plan for the future to identify stressors, build esteem and hope.
- Work with family/carers to solve problems, increase or maintain coping strategies.
- Develop structured, safe and meaningful daily activity.

---

principles of interventions discussed in relation to depression are also applicable here, with key points for management of self-harm summarized in Box 5.7.

Attention to delusional thinking and hallucinatory experiences is crucial in responding to the lived experience of the service user. Delusional thinking or recurring hallucinations can impact on the service user's level of hopelessness. Increased depressive symptoms have been associated with the perceived experience that a voice is omnipotent (Chadwick *et al.*, 1996), particularly when there is a sense of *no escape*. For example, where a person's ability to resist voices is poor, there may be an increased risk of self-harm (Fowler *et al.*, 1995).

It has also been argued that depression is a psychological reaction to having a debilitating condition like schizophrenia. This is akin to the grieving process where there is a reaction to loss of functions and status, similar to that experienced by others with severe disabilities. Recent advances in using cognitive therapy (similar to that used in depression) with people with schizophrenia have taken this view as a basis for intervention (Fowler *et al.*, 1995).

Violence or suicide attempts associated with schizophrenia (which may be precipitated by delusional thinking and hallucinations) can be a recurring risk for service users. Risk of relapse is also an important focus for nurses working with such people. Whilst it is widely agreed that individual experiences are unique, many people with schizophrenia will relapse. Taking antipsychotic medication does reduce this risk, but approximately 25% of service users with psychosis who are successfully maintained on medication will still relapse over a two-year period and as many as 40–60% over five years (Fowler *et al.*, 1995).

SOCIAL RISKS

One additional consequence of relapse is the risk of increasing social stigma and poor social skills. This refers to the negative impact of relapse on social roles and functions such as employment, relationships, networks, social skills and activities of daily living (Fowler *et al.*, 1995). Contributory factors can include chronic cognitive impairment, recurring acute episodes of psychosis, poor living and social situation, low self-esteem and poor outlook (Chadwick *et al.*, 1996; Fowler *et al.*, 1995; Gournay, 1996; Provencher *et al.*, 1997). In combination, these can lead to increased vulnerability and risk of self-neglect for individuals with schizophrenia (Neuchterlein *et al.*, 1994). Ignoring this risk can increase the likelihood of violent or self-harming events. Nevertheless, crises associated with homelessness, abuse, assault and poor physical health are also experienced by people with schizophrenia. Family support and psychoeducational, client-oriented, psychological interventions have been advocated as a means of improving overall social functioning (Fowler *et al.*, 1995).

Two key areas of intervention have been identified which aim at reducing these risks. First, psychoeducation covers information on psychotic symptoms and their management in addition to providing information on actions and effects of medication. This approach aims to improve self-management by the service user, family dynamics and successful access to the appropriate services (Falloon *et al.*, 1993; Gamble & Brennan, 1997). Secondly, cognitive behavioural therapy (CBT) provides tailored therapeutic strategies via individualized assessment and problem formulation. A psychotherapeutic approach is adopted where the service user's subjective experience of schizophrenia is the primary focus. Rather than rely on the illness model, the focus is on the service user's language and terminology. 'In such cases the aim is often to develop a good enough set of self-regulatory strategies to manage relapse' (Fowler *et al.*, 1995, p.13.)

Mental health nurses are increasingly incorporating CBT and psychotherapeutic approaches into their work with service users. However, it should be stressed that appropriate training in such techniques is essential. Nevertheless, the good practice aspects of individualized client-oriented interventions, with a focus on exploring the lived experience of symptoms, should allow nurses to help service users to gradually take responsibility for self-exploration and building of self-esteem.

ADDITIONAL RISKS

Non-compliance in taking antipsychotic medication has been linked to readmission (Day *et al.*, 1995) and to violent episodes (Steering Committee of the Confidential Inquiry into Homicides and Suicides by Mentally Ill People, 1996). The role of mental health nurses is to support service users to optimize control over their drug regimes (Gournay, 1996). This area of risk and nursing intervention is discussed in more detail in other chapters in this book.

NEW APPROACHES TO REDUCING RISKS IN SCHIZOPHRENIA

Recent developments in psychosocial approaches to working with people with schizophrenia are showing positive outcomes. Mental health nurses have begun to take a lead role in working with families in this way to reduce risk. These approaches have a problem-solving and supportive theme which includes systematic assessment and the use of cognitive behavioural approaches to underpin interventions. They encourage service user participation, include regular reviews and incorporate clinical supervision for staff carrying out the interventions.

It has been suggested that working with families may help reduce risks of violence to self or others by enabling them to examine negative behaviours towards each other. Models of educational support regarding trigger events and the impact of delusional thinking or hallucinations can encouraging openness and reduce high expressed emotion. It also recognizes the role and burden of the family and others who are significant to the service user. Awareness and acknowledgement of the individual experiences of schizophrenia may also increase family motivation to provide support. Additionally, provision of information regarding types of service and access, particularly outside office hours, may decrease feelings of isolation and improve overall family support mechanisms (Fowler *et al.*, 1995; Gamble & Brennan, 1997).

The psychological perspective to working with psychotic people is underpinned by the vulnerability–stress model (Neuchterlein *et al.*, 1994; Provencher *et al.*, 1997) which focuses on the individual level of vulnerability and impact of environmental stress. Given a range of information-processing deficits, it proposes that interventions are made to act as buffers to stress. Interventions can range from skills training or psychosocial interventions to drug treatments (Fowler *et al.*, 1995; Provencher *et al.*, 1997). The argument here is that understanding the possible causes and the range of symptoms experienced by people with schizophrenia are important areas of knowledge and skill for those working with service users. It can help to reduce risks through improving the quality of life since the focus is on the person's lived experience and their psychological processes for coping with stresses associated with schizophrenia.

Recently, evidence has begun to emerge from controlled studies on the impact of this work on a range of risks and symptoms of schizophrenia including the risk of relapse, compliance with medication, self-care, social skills and substance abuse (Garrety *et al.*, 1997; Tarrier, 1997).

The initial findings on combined treatment programmes for psychotic illnesses support the view that benefits can be gained from validating an individualized rather than a disease model of care. Nevertheless, this does not mean that the very real experiences of the symptoms should be negated, but that a new paradigm approach could cover both perspectives by paying attention to the reduction of symptoms (through recognizing and acknowledging them as lived experiences) and to the person's desires in terms of occupation and social networks.

Work by Fowler and colleagues (1995) argues for a broader perspective on schizophrenia.

Applying psychological theory directly to the attempt to understand psychotic symptoms has several advantages over attempts to understand the problems of people with psychosis solely in terms of disease entities or illness constructs ... rather than assuming that all psychotic symptoms arise as manifestations of a single biological disjunction ... those aspects of the experiences, beliefs and behaviours of people with psychosis ... may be more clearly identified.

(Fowler *et al.*, 1995, p.38)

Another viewpoint focuses on the voices heard by individuals and sharing of experiences by those who hear them. The Hearing Voices Network in the UK enables people who hear voices to come together. This is an emerging area of research and practice development and has stemmed from a series of studies carried out by Marius Romme in Holland (Romme, 1998). In one survey, Romme asked participants (identified following responses to a television request) about their voices and how they coped with them (Romme *et al.*, 1992). Consequently, Romme & Escher (1993) suggest that hearing voices should not be regarded solely as a symptom of mental illness since many people who hear voices are not regarded as mentally ill. Subsequent and more recent studies have resulted in the production of a voice hearer interview schedule – the Maastricht interview – which aims to improve coping mechanisms with the individual who is hearing voices. More recently, Coleman & Smith (1997) have produced a workbook to guide voice hearers and their supporters in understanding voice hearing and building personal coping mechanisms. The reader is referred to the recent work of Romme and of Coleman & Smith to gain a more detailed understanding of this area of practice.

Table 5.1		Old paradigm	New paradigm
Summary of emerging thinking on schizophrenia and psychotic illnesses	Focus	Disease	Service user experience
	Setting	Institutional care	Community care
	Carer	Formal/custodial	Formal/informal/supportive
	Treatment	Medicines	Combination therapies

CONCLUSION

Mental health nurses should recognize their qualities as good observers, communicators and negotiators in addition to their basic skills of demonstrating empathy, understanding and safety. These skills underpin the management of crisis events and are particularly important for managing an acutely disturbed person. They can be very effective in breaking through the confusion, fear and frustration of schizophrenia and in helping to clarify issues in a crisis situation (even if only momentarily) for a service user who may be agitated, threatening violence or self-harm. Additionally, nurses can develop their medication management, supportive and therapeutic skills to work in the longer term with service users and their families, thereby reducing the long-term risks associated with schizophrenia.

People's experiences of schizophrenia are very complex and varied and there is a wide range of possible interventions. Therefore, mental health nurses need to take pertinent information about schizophrenia from quality research and combine this with effective practice and treatment information. This capability will increase the likelihood that the service user's own experiences and their symptoms will be identified and managed effectively, thereby reducing the associated risks.

REFERENCES

Alberg, C., Hatfield, B. & Huxley, P. (eds) (1996) *Learning materials on Mental Health Risk Assessment.* Manchester: University of Manchester and Department of Health.

American Psychiatric Association (1987) *Diagnostic and Statistical Manual of Mental Disorders*, 3rd edn. Washington, DC: APA.

Birchwood, M., McGorry, P. & Jackson, H. (1997) Early intervention in schizophrenia (editorial). *British Journal of Psychiatry.* 170:2, 5.

Carpenter, W.T. & Buchanan, R.W. (1994) Medical progress: schizophrenia. *New England Journal of Medicine.* 330, 681–690.

Carson, D. (1996) Risking legal repercussions. In: H. Kemshall & J. Pritchard (eds) *Good Practice in Risk Assessment and Risk Management*, Volume 1. London: Jessica Kingsley Publishers, pp. 3–12.

Chadwick, P., Birchwood, M. & Trower, P. (1996) *Cognitive Therapy for Delusions, Voices and Paranoia.* Chichester: John Wiley.

Coleman, R. & Smith, M. (1997) *Working with Voices: Victim to Victor.* London: Handsell Publications.

Dawson, P.J. (1997) A reply to Kevin Gournay's 'Schizophrenia: a review of the contemporary literature and implications for mental health nursing theory, practice and education'. *Journal of Psychiatric and Mental Health Nursing.* 4:1, 1–7.

Day, J.C., Wood, G., Dewey, M. & Bentall, R.P. (1995) A self-rating scale for measuring neuroleptic side effects. *British Journal of Psychiatry.* 166:5, 650–653.

Department of Health (1995) *Building Bridges: A Guide to Arrangements for Interagency Working for the Care and Protection of Severely Mentally Ill People.* London: HMSO.

Falloon, I.P.H., Laporta, M., Fadden, G. & Graham-Hole, V. (1993) *Managing Stress in Families.* London: Routledge.

Fowler, D., Garrety, P. & Kuipers, E. (1995) *Cognitive Behaviour Therapy for Psychosis: Theory and Practice*. Chichester: John Wiley.

Gamble, C. & Brennan, G. (1997) Working with informal carers and families of schizophrenia sufferers. In: B. Thomas, S. Hardy & P. Cutting (eds) *Stuart and Sundeen's Mental Health Nursing: Principles and Practice*. London: Mosby, pp. 487–504.

Garrety, P., Kuipers, E., Fowler, D. *et al.* (1997) A randomised controlled trial of cognitive behaviour therapy for psychosis. Paper presented at the Psychological Treatments for Schizophrenia Conference, Oxford, October.

Gelles, R. (ed) (1987) *Family Violence*, 2nd edn. London: Sage.

Gottleib, P., Gabrielson, G. & Kramp, P. (1987) Psychotic homicides in Copenhagen from 1959 to 1988. *Acta Psychiatrica Scandinavica*. 76:1, 285–292.

Gournay, K. (1996) Schizophrenia: a review of contemporary literature and implications for mental health nursing theory, practice and education. *Journal of Psychiatric and Mental Health Nursing*. 3:1, 7–12.

Hirsch, S. & Weinberger, D. (1995) *Schizophrenia*. Oxford: Blackwell.

Hogman, G. & Meier, R. (1995) *One in Ten: A Report by the National Schizophrenia Fellowship into Suicide and Unnatural Deaths Involving People with Schizophrenia*. London: National Schizophrenia Fellowship.

Link, B., Andrews, H. & Cullen, F. (1992) The violent and illegal behaviour of mental patients reconsidered. *American Sociological Review*. 57, 275–292.

Lipsedge, M. (1995) Clinical risk management in psychiatry. In: C. Vincent (ed) *Clinical Risk Management*. London: BMJ Books, pp. 277–293.

McGorry, P.D., Edwards, J., Mihalopoulour, C., Harrigan, S.M. & Jackson, H.J. (1996) EPPIC: an evolving system of early detection and optimal management. *Schizophrenia Bulletin*. 22:2, 305–326.

McNeil, T.F., Cantor-Graae, E., Nordstrom, L.G. & Rosenhind, T. (1993) Head circumference in 'preschizophrenic' and control neonates. *British Journal of Psychiatry*. 162, 517–523.

Monahan, J. (1988) Risk assessment of violence among the mentally disordered: generating useful knowledge. *International Journal of Law and Psychiatry*. 11, 249–257.

Monahan, J. (1992) Mental disorder and violent behaviour: perceptions and evidence. *American Psychologist*. 47:4, 511–521.

Monahan, J. & Steadman, H. (1983) Crime and mental disorder: an epidemiological approach. In: M. Tonry & N. Morris (eds) *Crime and Justice: An Annual Review of Research, Volume 4*. Chicago: Chicago University Press, pp.145–189.

Monahan, J. & Steadman, H.J. (eds) (1994) *Violence and Mental Disorder: Developments in Risk Assessment*. Chicago: University of Chicago Press.

Morgan, H.G. & Owen, J.H. (1990) *Persons at Risk of Suicide: Guidelines on Good Clinical Practice*. London: Boots Pharmaceuticals.

Neuchterlein, K.H., Dawson, M.E., Ventura, J. *et al.* (1994) The vulnerability–stress model of schizophrenic relapse: a longitudinal study. *Acta Psychiatrica Scandinavica*. 89, 58–64.

Provencher, H.L., Fournier, J.P. & Dupuis, N. (1997) Schizophrenia: revisited. *Journal of Psychiatric and Mental Health Nursing*. 4:4, 275–285.

Romme, M.A. (1998) *Understanding Voices: Coping with Auditory Hallucinations and Confusing Realities*. London: Handsell Publications.

Romme, M.A. & Escher, S. (1993) *Accepting Inner Voices*. London: MIND.

Romme, M.A., Honig, A., Noorthoorn, E.O. & Escher, S. (1992) Coping with hearing voices: an emancipatory approach. *British Journal of Psychiatry*. 161, 99–103.

Ryan, T. (1996) Risk management and people with mental health problems. In: H. Kemshall & J. Pritchard (eds) *Good Practice in Risk Assessment and Risk Management*, Volume 1. London: Jessica Kingsley Publications, pp. 93–108.

Steering Committee of the Confidential Inquiry into Homicides and Suicides by Mentally Ill People (1996) *Report of the Confidential Inquiry into Homicides and Suicides by Mentally Ill People*. London: Royal College of Psychiatrists.

Stuart, G.W. & Sundeen, S.J. (1995) *Principles and Practice of Psychiatric Nursing*, 5th edn. St Louis: Mosby.

Swanson, J.W., Holzer, C.E., Ganju, V.K. & Jono, R.T. (1990) Violence and psychiatric disorder in the community: evidence from the epidemiological catchment area surveys. *Hospital and Community Psychiatry*. 41, 761–770.

Takei, N., Sham, P.C., O'Callaghan, E. *et al.* (1994) Prenatal exposure to influenza and the development of schizophrenia: Is the effect confined to females? *American Journal of Psychiatry*. 152:1, 150–151.

Tarrier, N. (1997) Coping and problem solving in the treatment of persistent psychotic symptoms. Paper presented at the Psychological Treatments for Schizophrenia Conference, Oxford, October.

Taylor, P.J. (1985) Motives for offending among violent and psychotic men. *British Journal of Psychiatry*. 147, 491–498.

Taylor, P.J. (1995) Schizophrenia and the risk of violence. In: S. Hirsch & D. Weinberger (eds) *Schizophrenia*. Oxford: Blackwell, pp. 45–66.

Taylor, P.J. & Gunn, J. (1984) Violence and psychosis (1). Risk of violence among psychotic men. *British Medical Journal*. 288, 1945–1949.

Thomas, B., Hardy, S. & Cutting, P. (1997) *Stuart and Sundeen's Mental Health Nursing: Principles and Practice*. London: Mosby.

Wessely, S. (1997) The epidemiology of crime, violence and schizophrenia. *British Journal of Psychiatry*. 170 (supplement 32), 17–21.

Whittington, R. (1994) Violence in psychiatric hospitals. In: T. Wykes (ed) *Violence to Health Care Professionals*. London: Chapman & Hall, pp. 23–43.

Woodley, L., Dixon, K., Lindow, V. *et al.* (1995) *The Woodley Team Report of the Independent Review Panel to East London and the City Health Authority and Newham Council Following a Homicide in July 1994 by a Person Suffering with Severe Mental Illness*. London: East London and the City Health Authority and Newham Council.

World Health Organization (1992) *The ICD-10 Classification of Mental and Behavioural Disorders*. Geneva: WHO.

6 MANIC DEPRESSION: NURSING MANAGEMENT OF CRISIS AND RISK

Paul Needham

INTRODUCTION

Experiencing emotional ups and downs is part of the human condition. When these ups and downs are exaggerated, the consequences can be devastating in terms of misery, chaos, broken lives and suicide. Most of us can understand and empathize with the person who feels depressed when faced with failure or loss or feels excited on receiving good news or success. It is perhaps more difficult to fathom the violent mood swings that appear to affect more than 1% of the population (Jamison, 1995).

The physicians of ancient Greece noted this disorder 2000 years ago (Jackson, 1986) and the adoption of mental illnesses under a medical umbrella since the mid-19th century has seen the classification of this particular phenomenon under a variety of names including manic depression and bipolar disorder (Goodwin & Jamison, 1990).

People who are so labelled are in exalted company; among them are some of the most creative and prolific artists including Vincent van Gogh, Ernest Hemingway and Peter Tchaikovsky, who are understood to have taken their own lives, and Joseph Conrad, Robert Schumann, Edgar Allan Poe and Paul Gauguin who attempted suicide but did not succeed. It must be pointed out that these people experienced other physical and social problems that often seem to accompany manic depression. Thankfully, many talented people with manic depressive disorder did not succumb to their despair in this way. At the time of writing, Peter Gabriel, Spike Milligan, Axl Rose and Robin Williams, all of whom have publicly declared their manic depression, are still alive (names taken from Jamison, 1993). This list is not comprehensive and one does not need to have a mood disorder in order to be exceptionally creative; nor do mood disorders need hosts who are thus gifted since the majority of sufferers are not. Nevertheless, Jamison (1993) notes from past studies that a far higher number of established artists are diagnosed with manic depression or major depression according to the *Diagnostic and Statistical Manual of Mental Disorders (DSM-IV)* (American Psychiatric Association [APA], 1994a). This disproportion, Jamison suggests, may be the result of the increased energy, the bold and restless attitudes, the depth and variety of emotions and the expansive yet focused thought processes that are associated with hypomania, a state that lies somewhere between chaotic mania and normal mood.

Manic depression involves periods of mania, periods of depression and relatively normal gaps in between. There is, however, enormous variability in the patterns of frequency, duration and severity of these mood states between individuals and it seems that the only consistent criterion for this diagnosis is that the sufferer must have shown evidence of both mood extremes some time in his or her life (APA, 1994b). While depression can be very debilitating and distressing for the service user, with well-documented risks of suicide and self-neglect, it is often the highly disrupting manic phase that causes the most concern for others and is more likely to lead to hospitalization (Needham, 1997). Both mood extremes call for effective, tailored treatment responses and careful, ongoing assessment and management of risk.

Following a string of incidents of harm perpetrated by mentally ill individuals on others (for examples, see Davies *et al.*, 1995; Ritchie *et al.*, 1994; Spokes *et al.*, 1988), the term *risk management* is often read as the management of threats of violence to the public, to relatives and to carers by people with serious mental illnesses, and possibly to themselves (Ryan, 1996). While these dangers do exist in relation to people with manic depression, the risks associated with mania, depression and the bits in between are often different and also include the possibility of damage to social relationships, financial affairs, the person's living environment, employment, liberty and general health. If these risks are to be reduced, a comprehensive understanding of risk factors, a continuous assessment of mood and painstakingly detailed contingency planning to cover all the mood phases are called for. This requires a high level of commitment from the service user, his or her 'significant others' (meaning close relatives and friends) and a wide range of caring, social and occupational contacts.

This chapter looks at the contribution of the mental health nurse in this process, concentrating mainly on responses to problems associated with the manic phase. Details of the problems of depression and the risk and crisis management pertinent to this phase are ably covered in Chapter 7.

DEFINITION

This disorder is characterized by swings between extremely high and extremely low moods. The exact intensity, duration and behavioural manifestations of these phases are very varied and often difficult to predict and the speed of change from one mood to another can vary widely too.

In the manic phase, the service user experiences euphoria or irritation, increased energy (with little need for sleep), excitement and a sense of invulnerability. He or she may engage in extravagant, disruptive and dangerous behaviour which may result in physical injury, pregnancy, debt, crime, conflict with others and ruined marital relationships – problems which have long-term implications for the service user's recovery and may contribute to subsequent periods of depression and low self-esteem (APA, 1994b; Beach *et al.*, 1990; Coryell *et al.*, 1993). These risks arise out of behaviours reflecting extreme optimism and poor judgement, sometimes accompanied by grandiose ideas of special powers and special connections with God, celebrities or political leaders. Such delusions may include paranoid feelings which make the service user suspicious of, and potentially dangerous towards, others. Visual and auditory hallucinations sometimes occur. The person may show evidence of rapid and incomprehensible speech as they attempt vainly to keep pace with flights of abruptly changing ideas. One service user said of his manic experience:

When I first start to go high, I feel as if I can literally fly. I suddenly have such clarity of thought and purpose, and total conviction in my own infallibility. My insights into social, political and financial matters seem so simple but inspired that I believe I have the means to solve all the world's problems. As my mania progresses my thoughts come too fast and I can feel myself being swept away by a whirlwind of fleeting thoughts, emotions and an underlying sense of panic.

Drug and alcohol misuse is also a common problem in mania and depression which blurs the clinical picture and creates additional problems (Ghadirian & Roux, 1995; Winokur *et al.*, 1995), including an increased risk of violent behaviour (Alberg *et al.*, 1996).

Left untreated, the manic phase can last for months (APA, 1992). Eventually the mood falls to normal levels and may quickly descend to depression. There is a tendency to see mania and depression as the opposing poles of a continuum (as the name 'bipolar' implies) but it has been recognized that there is a *mixed episode* or *dysphoric mania* where the service user is still excitable or agitated but at the same time feels depressed. At this time, there is a greater risk of suicide as the service user feels the despair, recognizes the chaos they have been caught up in and has the energy and motivation to act on suicidal thoughts (Kahn *et al.*, 1996; Palmer & Gilbert, 1997).

Manic depression is, for most people, a chronic or lifelong illness which afflicts equal numbers of men and women, usually striking before the age of 35 and accounting for between 30% and 40% of admissions to acute psychiatric hospitals (APA, 1994b; The New York Cornell Hospital Medical Centre [NOAH], 1996; Shepherd & Hill, 1996). Recent research has highlighted gene and neuro-transmitter anomalies (National Institute of Mental Health [NIMH], 1996) although it is widely thought to be triggered by a combination of inherited vulnerability and life stresses (APA, 1994b; Gournay & Ritter, 1996), often called the *stress–vulnerability model* of mental health problems (Onyett, 1992).

TREATMENT

The drug treatments for manic depressive illness generally employ three distinct schemes:

1. the mood stabilizers;

2. the adjunctive medication for use in manic or depressed phases selectively;

3. the antipsychotic drugs which are used when evidence of psychosis exists.

The mood stabilizers (lithium is the most common) are held to be effective in ameliorating mood extremes (APA, 1994b; Goodwin & Jamison, 1990; Hendrix,

1995) although Gitlin *et al.* (1996) and Solomon *et al.* (1995) found the relapse rates to be very high among manic depressive service users despite continuous maintenance treatment with these drugs. Nearly half of service users continue to have problems with their social, domestic and occupational functioning (Goldberg *et al.*, 1995). Nevertheless, current literature stresses the need for the service user to take prescribed medication regularly. Unfortunately, failure to comply with medication is a common problem (Guthiel, 1982; Jamison, 1991) which has been held responsible for relapse (Goldberg *et al.*, 1995). Possible reasons for this are denial that there is a problem, dissatisfaction with the delay in achieving results, the procedures for monitoring safe blood drug levels and blood cell anomalies (regular blood sampling) and the numerous side-effects that commonly accompany these drugs (Needham, 1997). Mental health nurses have a natural central role in monitoring, advising and encouraging the service user to take medications (Gournay, 1995). Any attempt at risk management will need to consider this area of treatment.

Recent developments in psychosocial interventions have focused on the identification of early warning signs (*prodromes*), the identification and avoidance of environmental triggers, increasing the service user's capacity to cope and providing support and education to service users and their families (Needham, 1997).

ASSESSING RISK

Reliance on the clinical judgement of mental health nurses and other health care professionals has not proved very accurate in predicting a person's suicide, self-harm or violence towards others (Alberg *et al.*, 1996). It is known that suicide poses a significant risk for people diagnosed with manic depression. Goodwin & Jamison (1990) suggest that suicide was the cause of death for about 25% of this group compared to 1% of people not previously diagnosed with mental illness, and up to 50% make at least one suicide attempt. Although the risk of suicide is much less in the manic phase, the danger of self-harm and violence arises from extravagant, disruptive and risky behaviour.

Risk cannot be seen purely as the probability of inflicting harm to self or others (despite the political motives for promoting risk management). Madcap behaviour during a manic episode can create havoc for the service user and their family that can have profound, negative, long-term consequences.

The weaknesses of using clinical judgement to predict risk include many personal biases and prejudices. This often highly subjective decision can be influenced by the clinician's attitudes about the gender, age, appearance, race, accent, education, occupation and dress of the service user. Even the presence of the 'patient' in the health care setting with a diagnostic label can radically alter the way they are seen and treated by others (Alberg *et al.*, 1996; Hayward & Bright, 1997). Certainly, patients are aware of the stigma attached to them and this often decreases their self-esteem and engagement with others (Link, 1987) and may result in maladaptive problem-solving styles (Hayward & Bright, 1997). Effective risk assessment still entails the nurse (and other clinicians) investigating the person's current mental state and environmental circumstances and weighing these up together with a number of actuarial factors associated with increased risk (Alberg *et al.*, 1996) in order to make decisions that will ultimately affect their care, supervision and autonomy.

These problems are compounded by the type II error or false-positive prediction. Given a choice between making a high-risk or a low-risk prediction, the high-risk prediction that leads to increased vigilance and a number of other precautions will always be the safer bet. If the person fails to create harm, this can be seen as the result of prudent clinical precautions. If the person does create harm then the prediction is immediately vindicated. In contrast, the low-risk prediction will always hold some chance of being proved dramatically wrong, with the possibility of the nurse (or other clinician) being blamed for exercising poor judgement. It is difficult to say how many false positives actually occur in clinical practice. Alberg *et al.* (1996) suggest that there are two false positives for every one correct prediction but there may be a much higher number of errors. This obviously has enormous implications for service provision in unnecessary admissions to inpatient facilities. Once an 'at risk' or 'dangerous' label has been applied to the service user, that person may be subjected to yet more institutional prejudice, even when the factors which influenced this judgement have changed. Young age, for example, is an actuarial factor for increased risk of violence but as the service user grows older, the risks can be expected to decrease. Similarly, a current diagnosis of mania coupled with evidence of alcohol misuse would indicate that the person is also at high risk of aggression and violence. One week later the person has reverted to a normal mood and has stopped drinking alcohol. The risk of harm to others is now reduced although the risk of suicide is significantly greater.

These examples highlight the need for continuous assessment of risk and awareness, of changing circumstances. One way of avoiding the impact of individual prejudices and allowing decision making that looks beyond the needs of one individual is to develop multiagency assessments of risk, with the participation of the service user and relatives as much as possible. This process obviously needs to be handled with some care and diplomacy, respecting the confidentiality of sensitive information. If handled well, the assessment can be a positive rehabilitation exercise, establishing achievable goals for the service user's reduction in risk.

RISK FACTORS

Table 6.1 (adapted from Alberg *et al.*, 1996) shows the demographic and individual factors associated with higher risks for harm to others and suicide. It would be difficult to attribute a specific level of importance to any of these factors but the interrelation between these factors and manic depressive illnesses can be worthwhile knowledge for mental health nurses.

Table 6.1

Risk factors for harming others and suicide

Risk factors	Harm to others	Suicide
Demographic factors		
Age	Younger	Older
Gender	Male	Male
Living arrangements	Insecure accommodation	Living alone
Occupation	Insecure employment	Unemployed or retired
Mental health	Psychotic depression	Depression
	Manic depression	Schizophrenia
	Schizophrenia	Chronic insomnia
	Paranoid psychosis	
Physical health		Poor health/terminal illness/pain
Alcohol or substance misuse	Yes	Yes
Relationships		Separated/divorced/widowed
Personal details		
History	(Of previous violence)	(Of suicide attempts)
Recency	Recent	Recent
Severity	Severe	Severe
Frequency	Frequent	Frequent
Pattern	Involving specifiç people, places, etc. Justifies attitudes and ideas	i.e. at end of a relationship
Ideation	Deprecates self and others Fantasies, anger, frustration	Deprecates self and others
Plan and intention	Yes	Yes

(Adapted from Alberg *et al.*, 1996)

CONSIDERATION OF RISK AND CRISIS IN PRACTICE

CASE STUDY 6.1

Helen is a 36-year-old woman who lives with her husband and two young daughters (aged nine and six) in a relatively affluent suburb of town. She has a history of manic depressive illness spanning 10 years. Over this time Helen has suffered from mania several times, necessitating her admission to an acute psychiatric ward. After about three weeks of manic behaviour, Helen's mood has waned (with the help of medication). On previous admissions, Helen's mania has been followed by depression which has lasted for between two and 10 weeks. It was during a spell of depression two years ago that Helen attempted suicide by taking an overdose of a toxic cocktail of drugs. But this time the anticipated depression does not seem to have materialized and Helen, who is engaging in ward groups and activities with modest enthusiasm, is keen to be discharged so that she can look after her family and help out at the local playgroup where she previously worked as a volunteer. Her husband is supportive but he says he needs to commit himself to his demanding executive job and he is unable to take time off to look after Helen. His earning capacity has been made more crucial because of huge debts that have resulted from Helen's reckless spending. He has been looking after the children with the help of Helen's mother, who lives on the other side of town.

Some issues for the mental health nurse
- What are the risks?
- What further information might be needed?

Short-term issues
- Is Helen hiding a depression?
- Might she be planning suicide?
- Is she taking her medication?
- Is she hoarding tablets in readiness for a suicide attempt?
- Are Helen's children at risk in any way?

Long-term issues
- Is there evidence of alcohol or drug misuse?
- What is the nature of Helen's financial problems?
- What other domestic and social problems are involved?
- How much support is available within the family?
- What impact does Helen's illness have on her status and self-esteem?

At this stage, the risks are not readily identified but there are a number of short-term and long-term issues that call for further investigation. Among the immediate, short-term concerns is Helen's current mental state. Her apparent recovery seems to contrast with previous patterns where she has shifted from mania to depression. Could she have depression which she has managed to conceal from the ward staff? What evidence might be available to confirm her depression? Although expressed feelings of depression is the main symptom, one might also expect to see disturbances in concentration and memory, a loss or gain in appetite, a marked loss or gain in sleep and various unexplained physical ailments. Helen's mood, her negative feelings about herself and her intentions might be disclosed to a key worker or case manager who is able to show empathy and employ active listening skills (Egan, 1990). The impressions of Helen's husband and mother might also be sought. It would be tempting to accept Helen's reports of her mood at face value, affording her credit for honesty and attempting to empower her. However, it should be remembered that suicide attempts by manic depression sufferers during the depressed phase are alarmingly common, with a higher incidence among women, and that mixed states (*dysphoric mania*), characterized by symptoms of both mania and depression, are particularly risky (Jamison, 1996).

Jamison (1996) writes: 'The most reliable method of preventing suicide in patients with manic-depressive illness is to diagnose it early and accurately, and to aggressively treat the underlying illness' (p.4).

Helen might not be taking her medication. Compliance with medication is a major problem and nursing staff should check that the prescribed medication is actually taken. The drugs routinely prescribed for manic depression are extremely dangerous if taken in large quantities and hoarding them in readiness for an intended overdose poses a real threat. This threat should be taken seriously since Helen has a prior history of overdose.

At ages nine and six, Helen's children are still dependent and vulnerable. Although we might assume that they are safe in the supervision of their father and grandmother, it is not known what the home conditions are like. Financial problems have been revealed but this could also extend to repossessed furniture, disconnected essential services or even homelessness. Parents who are service users have been known to withhold details about their illness, behaviour and living conditions for fear of losing their children (Alberg *et al.*, 1996). The children are at risk of neglect when Helen is ill and at times when she is the sole carer. They may also be at risk of abuse from Helen when she is suffering from mania, either directly from her impulsive behaviour or by allowing others to take advantage. There is also the possibility that Helen might attempt to kill her children before she takes her own life, so that they 'will be saved from a cruel and uncaring world'.

These risks may be compounded by any alcohol or illegal drug misuse. These circumstances might be usefully investigated by a social worker who can also look at the children's histories, and their school progress as well as the needs of Helen's husband and mother.

These investigations are crucial to the determination of risk probabilities. Scott (1977) writes:

It is the patience, thoroughness and persistence in this process [risk assessment] rather than any diagnostic or interviewing brilliance, that produces results. In this sense the telephone, the written request for past records, and the checking of information against other informants, are the important diagnostic devices.

(p.129)

There may be a tendency to look at the risks associated with Helen's discharge within a narrow *risk minimization* approach, largely in terms of the potential for causing death and destruction. The *risk-taking* approach, by contrast, is interested in the risks for the service user in terms of disempowerment, social disintegration and quality of life (Davis, 1996). There is an obvious paradox here in that by taking measures to limit risks of violence, Helen might be stripped of important liberties that are essential for her self-esteem and autonomy. In practice, it is hoped that decisions made about Helen's future would consider her own needs as a human being and ways in which she can be helped to fulfil her role within her family and the wider society.

This balance will be threatened if important decisions are taken remotely by people who are unaware of Helen's strengths, needs and aspirations. Public misconceptions of mental illness can lead to infringements of individual rights if allowed to unduly influence decisions (Alberg *et al.*, 1996). Conversely, the balance may also be jeopardized if those decisions are taken without due consideration of legal and professional demands and the welfare of others. It seems that a balance of views and values of a number of agencies, including those of Helen and her family, may be needed to arrive at fair and equitable decisions. There are obvious practical difficulties in achieving this level of consultation and co-operation among all interested parties, which may never be entirely satisfied given the universal demand and resource problems.

Helen's Care Programme Approach (Department of Health [DoH], 1990) key worker (who is likely to be her community mental health nurse) will be required to co-ordinate the involvement of care services and to facilitate an ongoing assessment of Helen's needs. This will also involve continuous assessment of risk based on changing domestic circumstances and clinical wellness. This process will be helped immensely by an intimate knowledge of Helen and her world and a close relationship born out of a respect for Helen as a person and the ability to use active listening skills (Burnard, 1997).

There are a number of issues that Helen and her key worker might tackle when she is well. Pollack (1995) claims that many manic depressive sufferers complain about the lack of information and practical advice given to them. Helen can be given information and she can be encouraged to seek help from other sources, such as the Manic Depression Fellowship. This may encourage Helen to comply with prescribed medication, limit alcohol consumption, avoid unwarranted medications, establish regular sleeping habits, eat sensibly and look after her general health, all of which might help to stave off relapse. Helen may also attend support groups where she is able to share her experiences with other sufferers and also learn from their experiences.

Helen might also be helped to look over her past history for common patterns and triggers of her mood changes. Sometimes the onset of mood changes can be associated with peculiar events such as pay bonuses or personal celebrations (APA, 1994b). Charting Helen's manic and depressive episodes against her significant life events and treatments (using a system described by Post et al., 1988) can help to generate hypotheses which can be reviewed in the light of future experience.

The mental health nurse might help Helen to monitor her mood fluctuations and to identify the early warning signs of impending relapse. A number of studies suggest that each manic depressive sufferer has a unique pattern of prodromes, such as sleep irregularities, heightened sensitivity or racing thoughts which can give 2–4 weeks' forewarning of relapse. Smith & Tarrier (1992) suggest that more than 85% of patients report these prodromal signs. The nurse, working closely with the service user and their family, is in an ideal position to help identify the particular 'relapse signature'.

As key worker, the nurse can work with Helen and her family to arrange ongoing support and supervision and to help make contingency plans in anticipation of future periods of illness; for example, how risks can be reduced in relation to reckless spending and neglect or abuse of the children. These measures will no doubt take careful thought but may have the added bonus of giving Helen a sense of control and added motivation to plan for her own illness.

CASE STUDY 6.2

Mark is a 22-year-old university student living in the halls of residence on campus. He was admitted to an acute psychiatric ward one year ago when he experienced a short manic phase of six days followed by a longer period of depression which lasted several weeks and culminated in him being discharged to his parent's home. On this occasion he was able to resume his studies without having to drop back, although additional work was involved. Mark has been referred by his general practitioner to the mental health team for an urgent assessment. The residence manager reports that Mark has been shouting and playing loud music during the night and many of the other students are worried about his behaviour and annoyed that he has caused so much disruption within the house. Mark looks wild and unkempt as he paces the house and talks rapidly, displaying 'flights of ideas'. His mouth is caked with dried spittle and he smells strongly of body odour. His room is strewn with books and papers and a computer has been dismantled. He is unable to answer questions coherently. Your arrival has aroused more interest from other residents who ask if Mark is all right.

Some issues for the mental health nurse
• What are the immediate risks?
• What additional information might be needed for a further assessment of risk?

Although Mark is young and male, these factors and any history of previous violence are irrelevant at this stage. Mark's primary risks come from his possible self-neglect and any irresponsible risk-taking behaviours he engages in while he is manic. Admission to an inpatient facility is almost inevitable but an investigation of background information will be useful in determining immediate and longer term risks and provide some damage limitation where necessary. This type of emergency is not uncommon among manic depressive sufferers. With greater experience and the involvement of supportive family members (or close others), sufferers like Mark may be admitted before the full-blown manic episode develops, thus limiting the danger of physical and environmental catastrophe.

While this scenario can be viewed as a 'crisis' requiring immediate intervention, it does not conform to Caplan's (1964) description of a crisis. Caplan suggests that a crisis occurs when a conflict or problem is perceived as threatening and not readily solvable by means of previously successful problem-solving methods. Mark is clearly in a potentially threatening situation and his usual capacity for solving problems has been diminished by his mental state. There is, however, some doubt that he *perceives* these problems as threatening. The ability to cope with new problems requires stable psychological functioning with a reasonable understanding of the problem situation, a minimum of emotional disturbance and an ability to draw on past experience of where effective strategies have been used. When the person is unable to cope effectively, uncomfortable emotions, such as anxiety, are aroused and cognitive capabilities are diminished (Walbert-Burgess, 1985).

Crisis intervention is usually a brief, home-based therapy that attempts to resolve immediate, anxiety-provoking problems by helping the service user adopt appropriate coping strategies. It is doubtful whether Mark understands his immediate problems in the same way as those around him. In this case, Mark's psychopathology has been instrumental in precipitating the crisis and prevents him from considering and using adaptive solutions. The mental health nurse's response at this time will be to ensure Mark's safety and to deal with the crises experienced by others as a result of Mark's condition. Later, Mark's ability to participate in crisis intervention activities will increase as his mania subsides, but the problem will have altered. The crisis then facing Mark will probably be his inability to deal with unpredictable mood changes and loss of control. There may also be a quagmire of problems brought about by earlier events.

The immediate precautions for reducing risks in the inpatient setting will be to:

- maintain Mark's safety by removing hazards, maintaining supervision and ensuring that there are adequate staff on hand to prevent any possible harm to Mark or others if it becomes necessary;

- assist Mark to take medication which will help to reduce his activity levels;

- promote rest by reducing background stimulation but provide suitable physical activities as an outlet for frustration if necessary;

- use a calm but firm approach that establishes clear boundaries on acceptable behaviour;

- encourage Mark to take high-protein food and drinks regularly.

While the ward nurses are thus engaged, the social worker may wish to contact Mark's parents to inform them of his circumstances and to gain some background information on his current financial and domestic circumstances, his current relationships and details of his previous history (including incidents of violence and suicide attempts). The social worker may also wish to contact Mark's friends on campus for a picture of his past and recent behaviour, looking for evidence of reckless behaviour and damage. Mark's alcohol and drug intake will also be important as this will alter the clinical picture and may add to the potential for violent behaviour. The residence manager and course lecturer may also be contacted for information. The ward staff might be asked to take note of Mark's visitors as potential informants. Care needs to be taken to preserve confidentiality throughout the information-gathering process.

As Mark recovers, the process of risk assessment and management will be similar to that discussed for Helen:

- Calculate the suicide risk.
- Clarify current and future support networks.
- Identify ongoing financial and domestic problems.
- Educate about medications to maximize compliance.
- Involve Mark's parents in his recovery.

- Educate those involved about manic depressive illness and self-management.
- Discuss future academic and employment plans.
- Develop contingency plans for damage limitation in future episodes of illness.
- Identify patterns of mood change and possible triggers.
- Identify prodromes of relapse.

Conclusion

The person with manic depressive illness poses considerable challenges to mental health nurses wishing to predict risk and respond to crisis. The risks are considerable, but they vary in their nature depending on the phase of the illness. Because the behaviours associated with this condition are so varied, the application of actuarial risk factors is only one small part of a patchwork quilt, with the person's mental state, history and expressed intentions providing the main clues. An understanding of the specific risks associated with manic depression will be helpful, along with experience. This will not eliminate the problems of being overly cautious, being constrained by service resource deficiencies or jeopardizing the person's natural rights but this would be asking too much. It would be so much easier if the degree of a particular risk could be calculated mathematically but the formula still relies heavily on experience and clinical judgement.

Current literature suggests that black and white judgements about risk are not helpful or appropriate (for example, Alberg *et al.*, 1996) but the assessment of risk, especially as defined within the narrow risk minimization approach (Davis, 1996) usually follows questions such as 'Should this person be discharged from hospital?' or 'Is this person suitable for this residential care setting?'. In such cases the answer is either 'yes' or 'no' and the people charged with making this decision are likely to be bombarded with professional, moral and political dilemmas.

As a lecturer engaged in the training of student nurses, I can anticipate the primary concern of most students – 'Am I in any personal danger?', I suspect that this is also the overriding question silently posed by everyone with a healthy sense of self-preservation. Personal dangers do exist for mental health nurses working with manic depressive service users, as they do when nursing people with other types of mental illness. Consequently, I would offer the following, albeit brief, advice:

- always treat the service user with respect and sincerity;
- make it your business to investigate the risks associated with the individuals with whom you are dealing;
- foster a climate of support amongst your colleagues;
- make yourself familiar with the policies and procedures for dealing with violence;
- take every opportunity to attend appropriate training on managing aggression and violence;

- use every incident as a learning opportunity;
- spare a thought for other hapless people who often have to endure the same threats but for longer;
- don't take unnecessary risks.

REFERENCES

Alberg, C., Hatfield, B. & Huxley, P. (eds) (1996) *Learning Materials on Mental Health: Risk Assessment.* Manchester: Manchester University and Department of Health.

American Psychiatric Association (1992) *Manic Depressive/Bipolar Disorder.* Washington, DC: APA. (Internet source: [http://www.psych.org/public_info/MANIC-1.htm] 24th October 1997)

American Psychiatric Association (1994a) *Diagnostic and Statistical Manual of Mental Disorders* (4th edn). Washington DC: APA.

American Psychiatric Association (1994b) Bipolar disorder. *American Journal of Psychiatry.* 151:12, 2–36.

Beach, S.R.H., Sandeen, E.E. & O'Leary, K.D. (1990) *Depression in Marriage.* New York: Guilford Press.

Burnard, P. (1997) Helping people in crisis. *Journal of Community Nursing.* 11:8, 4–8.

Caplan, G. (1964) *Principles of Preventive Psychiatry.* New York: Basic Books.

Coryell, W., Scheftner, W., Keller, E.J., Maser, J. & Klerman, G.L. (1993) The enduring psychosocial consequences of mania and depression. *American Journal of Psychiatry.* 150:5, 720–727.

Davies, N., Lingham, R., Prior, C. & Sims, A. (1995) *Report of the Inquiry into the Circumstances Leading to the Death of Jonathan Newby (a Volunteer Worker) on 9th October 1993 in Oxford.* Oxford: Oxfordshire Health Authority.

Davis, A. (1996) Risk work and mental health. In: H. Kemshall & J. Pritchard (eds) *Good Practice in Risk Assessment and Risk Management*, Volume 1. London: Jessica Kingsley Publications. pp.109–120.

Department of Health (1990) *The Care Programme Approach for People with Mental Illness Referred to the Specialist Psychiatric Services.* London: DoH.

Egan, G. (1990) *The Skilled Helper: A Systematic Approach to Effective Helping*, 4th edn. Pacific Grove, California: Brooks/Cole.

Ghadirian, A.M. & Roux, N. (1995) Prevalence and symptoms at onset of bipolar illness among adolescent inpatients. *Psychiatric Services.* 46:4, 402–404.

Gitlin, M.J., Swendsen, J., Heller, T.L. & Hammen, C. (1996) Relapse and impairment in bipolar disorder. *American Journal of Psychiatry.* 152:11, 1635–1640.

Goldberg, J.F., Harrow, M, & Grossman L.S. (1995) Course and outcome in bipolar affective disorder: a longitudinal follow-up study. *American Journal of Psychiatry.* 152:3, 379–384.

Goodwin, F.K. & Jamison, K.R. (1990) *Manic Depressive Illness.* New York: Oxford University Press.

Gournay, K. (1995) Mental health nurses working purposefully with people with serious and enduring mental illnesses: an international perspective. *International Journal of Nursing Studies.* 32:4, 341–352.

Gournay, K. & Ritter, S. (1996) The nurse's support role. *Nursing Times.* 92:26, 44–45.

Guthiel, T.G. (1982) The psychology of pharmacology. *Bulletin of the Menninger Clinic.* 46:4, 321–330.

Hayward, P. & Bright, J.A. (1997) Stigma and mental illness; a review and critique. *Journal of Mental Health.* 6:4, 345–354

Hendrix, M.L. (1995) *Bipolar Disorder.* Rockville, Maryland: National Institute of Mental Health. NIH Publication No. 95-3679. (Internet source [http://www.bucksworld.com/bipolar-nimh.html] 11th March 1998)

Jackson, S.W. (1986) *Melancholia and Depression; From Hippocratic Times to Modern Times.* New Haven: Yale University Press.

Jamison, K.R. (1991) Manic depressive illness: the overlooked need for psychotherapy. In: B.D. Beitman & G.L. Klerman (eds) *Integrating Pharmacotherapy and Psychotherapy.* Washington, DC: American Psychiatric Press.

Jamison, K.R. (1993) *Touched with Fire: Manic-depressive Illness and the Artistic Temperament.* New York: Macmillan Free Press.

Jamison, K.R. (1995) Manic-depressive illness and creativity. *Scientific American.* 272:2, 62–67.

Jamison, K.R. (1996) *Suicide and Manic-depressive Illness.* New York: American Foundation for Suicide Prevention. (Internet source [http://www.afsp.org/research/jamison.html] 24th October 1997)

Kahn, D.A., Carpenter, D., Docherty, J.P. & Frances, A. (1996) *The Expert Consensus Guideline Series: Treatment of Bipolar Disorder.* Independence, Virginia: Expert Knowledge Systems.

Link, B.G. (1987) Understanding labelling effects in the area of mental disorders: an assessment of the effects of expectations of rejection. *American Sociological Review.* 52:1, 96–112.

National Institute of Mental Health (1996) *Scientists Close in on Multiple Gene Sites for Manic Depressive Illness.* Rockville, Maryland: NIMH Pendulum Resources Newswire. (Internet source [http://www.pendulum.org/articles/mult_gene_sites.htm] 11th March 1998)

Needham, P. (1997) What nurses can do to help. In: V. Varma (ed) *Managing Manic Depressive Disorders.* London: Jessica Kingsley Publications. pp. 82–99.

NOAH (The New York Cornell Hospital Medical Centre) (1996) *Fact Sheet: Bipolar Disorder (Manic-depressive Illness).* New York: NOAH. (Internet source [http://www.noah.cuny.edu/illness/mentalhealth/cornell/conditions/bipol.html] 24th October 1997)

Onyett, S. (1992) *Case Management in Mental Health.* London: Chapman & Hall.

Palmer, A. & Gilbert, P. (1997) What psychologists can do to help. In: V. Varma (ed) *Managing Manic Depressive Disorders.* London: Jessica Kingsley Publications, pp. 42–61.

Pollack, L.E. (1995) Treatment of inpatients with bipolar disorders: a role for self-management groups. *Journal of Psychosocial Nursing.* 33:1, 11–16.

Post, R.M., Roy-Byrne, P.P. & Uhde, T.W. (1988) Graphic representation of life course of illness in patients with affective disorder. *American Journal of Psychiatry.* 147:7, 844–848.

Ritchie, J., Dick, D. & Lingham, R. (1994) *The Report of the Inquiry into the Care and Treatment of Christopher Clunis.* London: HMSO.

Ryan, T. (1996) Risk management and people with mental health problems. In: H. Kemshall & J. Pritchard (eds) *Good Practice in Risk Assessment and Risk Management*, Volume 1. London: Jessica Kingsley Publications. pp. 93–108.

Scott, P.D. (1977) Criminal dangerousness and its assessment. *British Journal of Psychiatry.* 131:8, 127–142.

Shepherd, G. & Hill, R.G. (1996) Manic depression: do people receive adequate support? *Nursing Times.* 92:26, 42–44.

Smith, J.A. & Tarrier, N. (1992) Prodromal symptoms in manic depressive psychosis. *Social Psychiatry and Psychiatric Epidemiology.* 27:5, 245–248.

Solomon, D.A., Keitner, G.I., Miller, I.W., Shea, M.T. & Keller, M.B. (1995) Course of illness and maintenance treatment for patients with bipolar disorder. *Journal of Clinical Psychiatry.* 56:1, 5–113.

Spokes, J., Pare, M. & Royle, G. (1988) *Report of the Committee of Inquiry into the Care and After-care of Sharon Campbell.* London: HMSO.

Walbert-Burgess, N. (ed) (1985) *Psychiatric Nursing in the Hospital and the Community*, 4th edn, New Jersey: Prentice-Hall.

Winokur, G., Coryell, W., Akiskal, H.S. *et al.* (1995) Alcoholism in the manic-depressive (bipolar) illness: familial illness, course of illness, and the primary-secondary distinction. *American Journal of Psychiatry.* 152:3, 365–372.

7 CRISIS AND RISKS ASSOCIATED WITH DEPRESSION

Siobhan Sharkey

INTRODUCTION

While every crisis arguably involves some risks, issues around risk awareness and management do not solely relate to crisis events. One model of crisis intervention acknowledges the importance of balance and equilibrium in successful crisis resolution (Aguilera & Messick, 1990) and this is akin to the weighing up of options along the decision trail of risk management (Sharkey, 1997). Mental health nurses work with service users in a range of settings and roles. Many of their interventions relating to risks can feel directive and controlling to both the service user and the nurse (Muir-Cochrane, 1996). On this point it is worth remembering that the essence of being human is having choices and mental health nurses have a key responsibility to facilitate choice. This need not be contrary to risk management.

This chapter examines crisis and risks relating to depression and attempts to acknowledge the reality of the often direct and controlling way in which nurses intervene while at the same time encouraging the principle of choice whenever possible. There is a wide range of risks which depressed people face but the two most significant are suicide and self-harm. Therefore, this chapter will focus mainly upon these two areas. Additionally, a brief discussion at the end of the chapter summarizes work with three high-risk groups: women with postnatal depression, older people and children and adolescents. This discussion serves to point the reader towards a wider literature in these areas and selected further reading is also suggested at the end of the references.

THE NATURE OF DEPRESSION

Awareness of the various states of depression is necessary in order to be able to identify the very individual experiences, events and contexts which affect mood. A key skill for the mental health nurse managing risks related to depressive states is to be able to weigh up and make decisions with, and where appropriate on behalf of, service users in the light of changing mood and contexts.

Distinctions have been made between depressive syndromes, namely *endogenous* or *reactive* depressions, the former implying a disease process or biochemical imbalance within the central nervous system, the latter a human response process to external stressors. Distinctions have also been made between a dimensional view of depression and a categorical view (you have it or you don't) (Beck *et al.*, 1974; Gilbert, 1992). Either way, it is important for nurses to realize that experiences of depression from the sufferer's perspective vary greatly from one person to another and it is the experience which is central to the nursing focus.

Depression, from a dimensional perspective, can be seen to exist on a continuum of emotional responses or depressive states, from mild through to severe. The focus for mental health nurses is to support individuals within this continuum of responses and, increasingly, for the majority of nurses, this means towards the severe end of the continuum. Emotional states such as anger, joy or sadness are part of the normal human repertoire of responses to the world around us and the people within it – the stresses of everyday living. Absence of an emotional response to stress can in itself be regarded as abnormal since emotional responses help individuals react, adapt and move forward.

At the adaptive, or healthy, end (of the continuum) is emotional 'responsiveness'. This involves being affected by, and being an active participant in, one's internal and external worlds ... They are barometers that give a person feedback about himself and his relationships with others, and they help a person function more effectively in his world.

(Stuart & Sundeen, 1995, p. 438)

Through their training mental health nurses learn the array of medical diagnostic terms and descriptive categories of depression and associated disorders. The *Diagnostic and Statistical Manual of Mental Disorders (DSM III)* provides criteria for the diagnosis of major depression (simple or recurrent) and bipolar disorders (American Psychiatric Association [APA], 1987). In addition, the *International Classification of Diseases (ICD-10)* provides definitions for categories of mood disorders (World Health Organization [WHO], 1992). The reader is referred to these references for greater detail on medical diagnostic criteria.

Familiarity with the terms used to describe and classify depression and awareness of the biological and psychological theories of depression help nurses to identify and make decisions about service user needs. A good knowledge base is important for dealing with crisis or high-risk events when decisions may have to be made quickly. However, it should be the individual behaviours and experiences which influence decision making as far as possible. Characteristics of

---

Box 7.1

Theories and models of depression

- Genetic/biological: hereditary models or links to blood grouping
- Neurophysical: chemical changes
- Cognitive: negative evaluation of self
- Separation complex – grief/loss reaction
- Helplessness (learned) or hopelessness
- Inability to solve problems
- Environmental influences/behavioural interaction

severe or deep depression can include (but not exclusively) feelings of worthlessness, profound sadness and hopelessness. Anxiety states are also common in severe depression, along with agitation, irritability and hypochondrial preoccupation. In addition, the concept of hopelessness (the belief that wishes and desires will not be achieved) is regarded as a good indication of risk of suicide (Beck *et al.*, 1975). Theoretical approaches to understanding the causes of depression point to life or natural events (for example, seasonal affective disorder; see Rosenthal, 1993) and psychological reactions to them. From an individual's perspective, there are likely to be many life events and reactions which can lead to a depressed state.

RISK OF SUICIDE AND SERIOUS SELF-HARM

People with severe depression can become vulnerable to a range of social, environmental and physical changes, in addition to the very dangerous threats of serious self-harm or suicide. 'Any attempt to explain suicide must surely encompass at a pragmatic level all theoretical approaches – whether these be biomedical/interpersonal or social/environmental in nature' (Morgan & Owen, 1990, p.2).

However, not all suicides or suicide attempts are by individuals with a clinical diagnosis of depression. Stressful and negative life events can become triggers for suicidal ideation and attempts, such as drug or alcohol abuse. Other mental illnesses, such as schizophrenia, also carry a risk of suicide (Alberg *et al.*, 1996; Morgan, 1994).

Morgan (1994) lists the high-risk groups for depression that carry a 15% risk of suicide as:

- male;
- older;
- single;
- separated and/or socially isolated;
- previous deliberate self-harm with recurring insomnia, neglect or agitation.

Mental health nurses and multidisciplinary teams (MDT), in assessing the biological, social, psychological and economic problems in a person's life, also need to consider the issue of changing contexts and the changing potential of trigger events superimposed upon existing problems. These may also be experienced as recurring patterns which are woven into the ongoing life experiences of the person.

Self-harm and attempted suicide can be differentiated by cause and intent. For instance, self-harming behaviour does not automatically imply an intention to kill oneself (parasuicide), but may be used as a coping mechanism. While the means used, such as self-poisoning or self-inflicted physical injury, may be the same regardless of intent, nurses need to be aware of the differing psychological and social factors which lead to self-harm. Factors other than depression can lead to

---

Box 7.2

High-risk indicators for suicide

- Deliberate self-harm.
- Following admission to a mental health unit, particularly during the first week.
- Following discharge from a psychiatric setting, particularly during the first month.
- Drug or alcohol misuse.
- Recent major life event such as divorce or separation.
- Being from a particular occupational group, such as farmer or doctor, or being unemployed.
- Non-compliance with treatment/medication.
- Rapid change in treatment type or in accommodation setting.
- Poor relationships with carers.

(Adapted from Alberg *et al.*, 1996; Gunnell, 1994; Morgan & Owen, 1990; Thomas *et al.*, 1997)

---

self-harming behaviours; for example, anxiety, aggression, guilt and psychosis (Burrow, 1994).

In addition, approximately 1% of people who carry out an act of non-fatal deliberate self-harm will kill themselves within a year. Ten percent will kill themselves at some time in the future and previous attempts are regarded as a clear indication of future attempts particularly if the attempt:

- is premeditated and serious (e.g. suicide note or leaving a will);
- is in an isolated place;
- uses a violent method (e.g. gun, lethal drugs) (Morgan, 1994).

Supporting individuals towards positive thinking and positive behaviours is a challenging role for nurses (Long & Reid, 1996). Often mental health nurses are asked to care for people in institutional settings where support is, in part at least, restrictive and controlling. Furthermore, such environments can be contrary to a philosophy which increasingly aims to regard service users as equal partners in their care. Nevertheless, in weighing up the need to protect life and prevent harm while respecting the personal freedom of the person, the team must regularly and rigorously assess, with the service user wherever possible, the likelihood of future self-harm or suicide attempt and provide support in the least restrictive way possible. During crisis periods safety is obviously a priority, but it is important not to ignore other aspects of a person's life experience at such times. Therefore, maintenance of dignity and respect for the service user should also be key considerations.

Full assessment should gather information on:

- symptoms and their duration;
- psychological, environment and social stressors and their duration;
- any prior attempts at suicide or self-harm;
- social contexts of attempts;
- support networks (Lambert, 1994; Libberton, 1996; Ryan, 1996; Sharkey, 1997).

Furthermore, the potential range of experiences surrounding negative affect and hopelessness provide additional warning signals to the nurse regarding the possible immediacy and level of risks. For mental health nurses, awareness of these issues needs to be coupled with skills in assessing and managing both the short-term crisis and longer term risks, such as serious self-harm, physical deterioration, accidents and loss of relationships (Sharkey, 1997).

MANAGING RISK OF SUICIDE AND SELF-HARM

The high and dangerous (life-threatening) risks of suicide or serious self-harm are especially devastating for the service user, their family and friends, as well as the nurse involved in care. Mental health nursing skills of observation, questioning and relationship building revolve around the use of verbal and non-verbal communication. These skills are crucial when working with service users likely to be at high or immediate risk of suicide or serious self-harm due to depression. It is likely that in crisis situations, where time and safety are paramount, a nurse will have to make decisions about the level and immediacy of risk of suicide or self-harm without having an opportunity to discuss events with the service user or others. In these circumstances it is important to negotiate with the service user and discuss decisions with other members of the team wherever possible. All available information should be recorded immediately and communicated with the team and reviewed at agreed time intervals throughout periods of high risk, regardless of cause or intent. Self-rating scales and instruments administered by nurses or other professionals can be useful at these times (see Chapter 13).

Community management

As the central figure in successful community care, the mental health nurse needs to be confident that they have obtained information from a wide range of sources:

- interviews and discussion with the service user;
- interviews and discussion with the family and friends (where appropriate);
- use of rating scales;
- the experience of the MDT.

It is the ongoing assessment upon which decisions for longer term needs and risk of suicide are made, with safety of the individual always paramount.

A nurse may receive a direct referral from a GP and find themselves the only specialist professional or contact for a suicidal person in the community. If this occurs, it is important to alert the MDT at the earliest opportunity. If first contact is made in the community, the assessment by the mental health nurse may indicate that the person's suicide risk is high enough to warrant inpatient management. If this is the case the GP or psychiatrist (if they have one) should be informed and the normal processes of admission, whether on a voluntary or involuntary basis, should be followed. 'Community management is not indicated when there is a grave risk of suicide or lack of adequate support, or both, or failure to establish a good working alliance with the patient' (Lipsedge, 1995, p.227).

Monitoring of changes in mood and intent of self-harm or suicide are more difficult outside a mental health unit. Access to the means of self-harm is also less likely to be under the control of the nurse in a community setting. Consequently, a significant degree of responsibility and accompanying stress is placed on the service user. The usefulness of Roy's model in facilitating a stress reduction and problem-solving approach may provide a therapeutic framework for managing suicide risk in a community setting, helping the person to identify the experiences and settings which are sources of their stress. This allows the person to take control in a planned way. Setting the plan and identifying key stressors can become a focus for discussions with the nurse and can be used as an anchor for the first steps of building confidence and self-esteem. Achievements and positive events can be identified and used as reminders of progress by the service user. Giving a copy of the care plan to the service user can provide a tangible record of progress (Libberton, 1996; Roy, 1976).

In addition to aiming to keep a person safe in the community setting, the nurse should aim to build a relationship of trust. This can be achieved by providing verbal and non-verbal messages of warmth and caring. Active listening and empathic responses can provide support and encouragement. Reassurance that the person can have a future will also help build a therapeutic relationship. Using time together to gain additional information from the service user will help the nurse (and team) make decisions about safety in community settings. If a person is saying they want to die, gauging levels of intervention can be undertaken through asking questions such as: 'Have you thought how you might carry this out?' or 'Have you ever attempted this before?' or 'Are you able to stop yourself thinking about dying?'. The nurse should, however, be careful not to adopt constant questioning and should avoid being pushy in their approach. Rating scales may be useful in decision making about safety in the community and the nurse should consult colleagues whenever possible.

Use of the Care Programme Approach will help ensure appropriate treatment and support needs are met, as well as regular reviews. Optimizing the role of carers and use of community facilities will help maximize contact between service users and mental health professionals. Consequently, this will help to reduce the risks associated with isolation and neglect (Department of Health [DoH], 1996). A summary of key strategies is given in Box 7.3.

In addition, the nurse must be aware of the possibility of denial of intent or

---

Box 7.3

Key strategies for community care of high risk service users

- A systematic approach to care should be used. This can include planned visits by the mental health nurse or other professionals, matching/increasing frequency and therapeutic content of visits between the person and nurse. Use of regular day care may be considered.

- Rapid follow-up should take place if the person fails to keep an appointment or attend day care.

- Good liaison with primary health care team, particularly in relation to medication prescriptions (frequency in small doses). Good family contact, where appropriate, to support needs or access to services (24 hours).

---

shortlived improvement which may be the result of taking antidepressant medication. Mood can increase before suicide intention has decreased (Becker-Fitz, 1987). This is particularly important in community settings as access to means of suicide or self-harm is readily available. The nurse (and team) need to be aware of the continuing risk associated with recovering drive and motivation as depression lifts. The nurse must therefore be vigilant when visiting in the community for any possible signs of deepening depression and increasing signs of risk of suicide and self-harm. Any signs should be recorded and communicated to others involved in the care package.

The nurse should begin to build upon any initially established relationship. This should aim at focused problem solving with the service user and ultimately reduce the impact of stressors on them. The use of contracts has also been advocated with people living in community settings (Alberg *et al.*, 1996). They have been used to provide a way in to working with suicidal people, but they have been criticized on the basis that they may lead to a lowering of intervention, with undue reliance on the contract (Egan, 1997). Contracts in a community setting should therefore be used with clear supervision arrangements and in agreement with the whole MDT. Contracts have also been advocated as a means of reducing self-harming behaviours for reasons other than low mood. As with depression, it is important to identify with the person the times and circumstances which lead to self-harming along with alternatives to this (Burrow, 1994).

For people whose suicide intentions persist or recur, it is important that continued optimistic support is available. It is crucial that assessment is repeated by the nurse and communicated within the team. It is also important that family and friends of the person are involved in this process. If high risk of suicide is assessed, admission or readmission to hospital may be considered, perhaps under the Mental Health Act (1983). Close contact and continuous monitoring to identify any increased risk are therefore crucial with a severely depressed person living in the community.

Inpatient management

The period immediately after admission to hospital can be a time of increased risk. It is often at this time that service users are placed on continuous observation, with safety firmly at the centre of the management plan.

It is important that the reasons for continuous observations are shared with the service user in an unambiguous and sensitive way. Any intervention which threatens the service user's level of control over their own behaviour should be kept to a minimum. The need for constant observation (also known as one-to-one or high-intensity observation) should be regularly reviewed and negotiated (where possible) with the service user. Clear, accurate and legible record keeping is essential to ensure safety. It may also assist the nurse to account for their actions at a later point should the worst happen.

During one-to-one or high-intensity observation periods, the nurse undertaking the intervention needs to strive to provide therapeutic input. Nurses should not avoid asking direct questions of the service user about their intentions. When identifying the need for constant one-to-one observation, the nurse also needs to consider any known history, current behaviours, communications (verbal and non-verbal) and contexts which are affecting the service user. Vigilance in respect of the physical environment is also important. For example, if the service user is in a single room this will help maintain safety, although the nurse should be alert to the frustration that this could cause the service user. Access to windows and exits, as well as the strength of shower curtains and bed clothes, should be reviewed to ensure they do not constitute a means of committing suicide (Lipsedge, 1995). Additionally, it is the responsibility of the nursing team, and in particular the key worker, to identify and request adequate staffing levels to ensure safety on clinical areas. Any difficulties in obtaining identified staffing should be communicated to the department head or manager. Recurrent problems should be dealt with in writing as soon as possible as it may be regarded as negligent on the part of the team if problems in staffing are not resolved.

It may become necessary for a nurse and colleagues to physically restrain an actively suicidal person and this should also be carried out with minimal physical contact and sensitivity. Acknowledging the role of the service user throughout the physical intervention and returning control to them as soon as possible can help maintain and restore self-worth and dignity.

As in community settings, denial of intent is a possibility. The dangers of *malignant alienation* can occur where the service user is distanced from both staff and carers because of challenging behaviours or repeated relapses of suicide intent and attempts (Watts & Morgan, 1994). This can have lethal consequences as it prevents relationship building and may create opportunities for access to the means of suicide or self-harm.

Over time the priority of safety regimes lessens as suicide intent decreases. As in community settings, the nurse and team need to be aware of the continuing risk which accompanies recovering drive. The continued use of empathy to build an open and honest relationship will underpin this ongoing work.

As suicide intent recedes the service user may not need constant observation. It is important to involve the service user in any change aimed at reducing the level of observation undertaken and ensure that they understand what has been agreed. The service user should be made aware that intermittent observation will mean a nurse will seek them out at set periods of time or they should know what is expected if the responsibility is given to them to present to the nurse at agreed intervals. The intervals can be lengthened should this arrangement prove successful. This approach helps to maintain service user control. As soon as is therapeutically possible, the nurse should also begin to spend non-observation time with the person to provide consistency of interaction. This gives a message of care and interest to the user who may be susceptible to thoughts of low self-worth.

As with community nursing, thorough ongoing assessment and relationship building with the service user may be accompanied by goal setting and planning ahead. The nurse needs to be sensitive to changes in mood and behaviour throughout in order to help pace the ability of the person to make their plans. Ultimately, the nurse can support the service user in emotional expression. Exploration of interpersonal relationships and networks, identifying ways to enhance these and building esteem are all areas where the nurse can provide support.

The nurse will aim to support the service user in developing a positive self-image (building relationships and developing a sense of belonging) during leave or discharge preparation. The nurse should recognize the increased risk that separation can cause and needs to work closely with significant people, such as friends and family, who will provide informal support in addition to the mental health professionals who will support them in the community. Furthermore, the service user should be encouraged to telephone or return to the unit any time while on leave should they feel they have increasing feelings of suicide or self-harm (Lipsedge, 1995). It is particularly important to avoid isolation following discharge, particularly during the first month (Goldacre *et al.*, 1993), so discharge planning should be undertaken alongside the nurse who will be supporting the person in the community.

As with any difficult or high-risk area of care, supervision and support for staff are essential. This should be available both as ongoing clinical supervision and the opportunity to undertake critical incident reviews. Nurses can utilize their clinical supervision sessions to review and reflect on their practice in any high-risk area of care. Nurses can use supervision to explore their attitudes to a person in their care who wishes to end their life. Long & Reid (1996) suggest that nurses can have a positive attitude to caring for this group of service users. Nevertheless, frustration and rejection may be experienced by nurses and supervision offers an opportunity to reflect on those feelings (Hardy & Minghella, 1997).

POSTNATAL DEPRESSION

Depression following pregnancy and childbirth may also lead to thoughts of suicide, serious self-harm or harm to the baby.

Box 7.4

Causes and symptoms of postnatal depression

Causes
- Physical problems (of either the mother or baby during a difficult birth)
- Social factors (isolation, lack of family support, poor professional help)
- Psychological factors (loss of control, loss of esteem or confidence, problems with role changes and identity)

Physical and psychological symptoms
- Lack of sleep
- Loss of appetite
- Anxiety
- Feelings of paniç
- Confusion
- Obsessional thinking
- Fear of having the baby or profound sadness (can last for many months or even years following the birth)

(Adapted from Cox *et al.*, 1987; Gilbert, 1992; Littlewood & McHugh, 1997)

Postnatal depression can be defined as a first episode psychiatric illness occurring within the first six months of the baby being born, requiring professional help and support. Postnatal depression can be experienced on a scale ranging from 'postpartum blues' to moderate depression, to severe depression, to puerperal psychosis.

(Littlewood & McHugh, 1997, p.19)

The Edinburgh Postnatal Depression Scale is a useful self-report scale which, while not a predictor of depression, may provide a focus for the mother and nurse to begin to explore issues around the low mood (Cox *et al.*, 1987). As with other depressive illnesses, establishing a therapeutic relationship between the mother and nurse, in addition to supporting the family and significant others, is a key to rebuilding esteem and confidence. Littlewood & McHugh (1997) provide a good starting point for readers wanting a greater knowledge of this area.

OLDER PEOPLE

The *Health of the Nation Key Area Handbook - Mental Illness* (DoH, 1993) points out that while only 15% of the population is over 65, this group accounts for a quarter of all suicides. Physical, social and psychological theories of depression serve as causes for depression with older people, as with younger age groups. However, depression in older people can manifest in quite different ways from that of younger people. It is worth noting that loss and physical illness are more common experiences for older people and can be particular risk factors for this group. Losses in relation to health, employment, status, mobility, social support, visual and auditory senses, bereavement and independence are often experienced by older people and can lead to severe depression and suicide (Morgan & Owen, 1990). Ageism is a real risk when the view is held that the threat to life by suicide is not as important for older people because they are closer to the age of a natural death. This view negates the negative and distressing experiences often suffered by older people (Duffy, 1997).

Assessment is important with older service users as there is a risk of misdiagnosis due to similarity with physical problems common in this group. In addition, there may be overlaps between depressive symptoms and dementia or changes in eating, disturbed sleep patterns and paranoia. Involvement of other professionals and family will ensure a good breadth of information.

Careful listening to what older people say and observation of any changes in routine or patterns of behaviour may reveal increasing negative thinking. Changing a will, planning a funeral or an increase in motivation following severe depression may all be important suicide risk indicators. At these times, it is important to openly ask the person about their feelings and intentions. Readers are referred to Duffy (1997) and Lindesay (1991) for additional information on indicators of depression in older people.

CHILDREN AND ADOLESCENTS

Figures indicate that 10% of children have moderate or severe mental health problems with around 2% of children being depressed (Graham & Hughes, 1995). One Northern Ireland study shows an apparent increase in suicides by younger males aged 15–24, particularly using violent methods (McLaughlin & Whittington, 1996).

Causes of depression in children or adolescents are likely to be a combination of physical, psychological and social (particularly familial) conditions (Russell-Johnson, 1997). These may include physical illness and repeated hospital admissions, accidents, physical or sexual abuse, bullying, neglect, parental mental health problems or parental disharmony and isolation. Repeated fostering or prolonged institutional care and environmental conditions may also be linked to emotional problems in children (Barker, 1995; Pinto & Whisman, 1996; Thomas et al., 1997).

Experiences of loss and deprivation may lead to depression in children and adolescents. However, they may also lead to feelings of frustration and anger which can manifest in self-harming behaviours rather than suicidal ideation and attempts. Multiprofessional and multiagency working is particularly important with children and adolescents experiencing depression.

Nurses working with an actively suicidal adolescent should follow similar risk management to the processes already discussed. However, it has been suggested that adolescents have different needs from children and adults and are better cared for in peer groups or should at least have access to siblings or peers. Adolescents can respond positively and appear motivated while in hospital but this can rapidly drop once they leave hospital (Foote, 1997). Assessment should therefore be ongoing within the home setting until intent no longer exists.

CONCLUSION

Self-harming and suicidal behaviours associated with depression are encountered in both community and hospital settings by mental health nurses. Nurses may work with people in crisis or on a longer term basis and therefore require the knowledge and skills to prevent harm while understanding the person's perspective and wishes. Caring for this group of people is therefore difficult and can be emotionally draining as well as therapeutically challenging. A systematic approach through the effective use of assessment frameworks and multidisciplinary working which involves the service user are important aspects in the management of risks associated with depression.

REFERENCES

Aguilera, D.C. & Messick, J.M. (1990) *Crisis Intervention: Theory and Methodology.* St Louis: Mosby.

Alberg, C., Hatfield, B. & Huxley, P. (eds) (1996) *Learning Materials on Mental Health Risk Assessment.* Manchester: Manchester University and Department of Health.

American Psychiatric Association (1987) *Diagnostic and Statistical Manual of Mental Disorders*, 3rd edn. Washington, DC: APA.

Barker, P. (1995) *Basic Child Psychiatry.* Oxford: Blackwell Science.

Beck, A.T., Weissman, A., Lester, D. & Trexler, L. (1974) The measurement of pessimism: the Hopelessness Scale. *Journal of Consulting and Clinical Psychology.* 42:6, 861–865.

Beck, A.T., Kovacs, M. & Weissman, A. (1975) Hopelessness and suicidal behaviors: an overview. *Journal of the American Medical Association.* 234, 1146–1149.

Becker-Fitz, T. (1987) Keeping a suicidal patient safe while hospitalised. *Ohio Nurses Review.* 62:10, 6.

Burrow, S. (1994) Nursing management of self-mutilation. *British Journal of Nursing.* 3:8, 382–386.

Cox, J.L., Holden, J.M. & Sagousky, R. (1987) Detection of postnatal depression: development of the Edinburgh Postnatal Depression Scale. *British Journal of Psychiatry.* 130, 782–788.

Department of Health (1993) *The Health of the Nation: Key Area Handbook – Mental Illness.* London: HMSO.

Department of Health (1996) *Building Bridges: A Guide to Arrangements for Interagency Working for the Care and Protection of Severely Mentally Ill People.* London: The Stationery Office.

Duffy, D. (1997) Suicide in later life: how to spot risk factors. *Nursing Times.* 93:11, 56–57.

Egan, M.P. (1997) The 'no suicide contract': helpful or harmful? *Journal of Psychosocial Nursing*. 35:3, 31–33.

Foote, J. (1997) Teenage suicide attempts. *Nursing Times*. 93:22, 46–48.

Gilbert, P. (1992) *Depression: The Evolution of Powerlessness*. Hove: Lawrence Erlbaum.

Goldacre, M., Seagroatt, V. & Hawton, K. (1993) Suicide after discharge from psychiatric inpatient care. *Lancet*. 342(I), 283–286.

Graham, P. & Hughes, C. (1995) *So Young, So Sad, So Listen*. London: Gaskell & West London Health Promotion Agency.

Gunnell, D. (1994) *The Potential for Preventing Suicide: A Review of the Literature on the Effectiveness of Interventions Aimed at Preventing Suicide*. Bristol: Health Care Evaluation Unit, Bristol University.

Hardy, S. & Minghella, E. (1997) Understanding suicidal behaviour. In: B. Thomas, S. Hardy and P. Cutting (eds) *Stuart and Sundeen's Mental Health Nursing: Principles and Practice*. St Louis: Mosby, pp. 237–252.

Lambert, C. (1994) Depression (part 2): nursing management. *Nursing Standard*. 8:48, 57–62.

Libberton, P. (1996) Depressed and suicidal clients: how nurses can help. *Nursing Times*. 92:43, 38–40.

Lindesay, J. (1991) Suicide in the elderly. *International Journal of Geriatric Psychiatry*. 6:6, 355–361.

Lipsedge, M. (1995) Clinical risk management in psychiatry. In: C. Vincent (ed) *Clinical Risk Management*. London: BMJ Books, pp. 277–293.

Littlewood, J. & McHugh, N. (1997) *Maternal Distress and Postnatal Depression: The Myth of Madonna*. Basingstoke: Macmillan.

Long, A. & Reid, W. (1996) An explanation of nurses' attitudes to the nursing care of the suicidal patient in an acute psychiatric ward. *Journal of Psychiatric and Mental Health Nursing*. 3:1, 29–37.

McLaughlin, C. & Whittington, D. (1996) Suicide in Northern Ireland: A comparison of two quinquennia (1982–1986 and 1987–1991). *Journal of Psychiatric and Mental Health Nursing*. 3:1, 13–20.

Morgan, H.G. (1994) *Suicide Prevention: The Assessment and Management of Suicide – A Guide for Healthcare Professionals*. Norwich: Anglia University Press.

Morgan, H.G. & Owen, J. (1990) *Persons at Risk of Suicide: Guidelines on Good Clinical Practice*. London: Boots Pharmaceuticals.

Muir-Cochrane, E. (1996) Therapeutic interventions associated with seclusion of acutely disturbed individuals. *Journal of Psychiatric and Mental Health Nursing*. 3:5, 319–325.

Pinto, A. & Whisman, M.A. (1996) Negative affect and cognitive biases in suicidal and non-suicidal hospitalised adolescents. *Journal of the American Academy of Child and Adolescent Psychiatry*. 35:2, 158–165.

Rosenthal, N.E. (1993) Diagnosis and treatment of seasonal affective disorder. *Journal of the American Medical Association*. 270, 2717–2720.

Roy, C. (1976) *Introduction to Nursing: An Adaptation Model*. Englewood Cliffs, New Jersey: Prentice-Hall.

Russell-Johnson, H. (1997) Deliberate self-harm in adolescents. *Paediatric Nursing*. 9:1, 29–34.

Ryan, T. (1996) Risk management and people with mental health problems. In: H.

Kemshall & J. Pritchard (eds) *Good Practices in Risk Assessment and Risk Management,* Volume 1. London: Jessica Kingsley Publications. pp. 93-108.

Sharkey, S. (1997) Clinical risk and depression. *Nursing Standard.* 11:18, 47–55.

Stuart, G.W. & Sundeen, S.J. (eds) (1995) *Principles and Practices of Psychiatric Nursing,* 5th edn. St Louis: Mosby.

Thomas, B., Hardy, S. & Cutting, P. (eds) (1997) *Stuart and Sundeen's Mental Health Nursing: Principles and Practice.* London: Mosby.

Watts, D. & Morgan, H.G. (1994) Malignant alienation: dangers for patients who are hard to like. *British Journal of Psychiatry.* 164:1, 11–15.

World Health Organisation (1992) *The ICD 10 Classification of Mental Health and Behavioural Disorders.* Geneva: WHO.

SELECTED READING

Children and adolescents

Barker, P. (1995) *Basic Child Psychiatry.* Oxford: Blackwell Science.

Graham, P. & Hughes, C. (1995) *So Young, So Sad, So Listen.* London: Gaskell & West London Health Promotion Agency.

Russell-Johnson, H. (1997) Deliberate self-harm in adolescents. *Paediatric Nursing.* 9:1, 29–34.

Shapiro-Gottlieb, P. (1994) *A Parent's Guide to Childhood and Adolescent Depression.* New York: Bantam Doubleday Dell.

Weller, E. & Weller, R.A. (1991) Mood disorders in children. In: J. Wiener (ed) *Textbook of Child and Adolescent Psychiatry.* Washington, DC: American Psychiatric Press, pp. 167–175.

Postnatal depression

Ballard, C.G., Davis, R., Cullen, P.C., Mohan R.N. & Dean, C. (1994) Prevalence of postnatal psychiatric morbidity in mothers and fathers. *British Journal of Psychiatry.* 164: 782–788.

Cox, J.L., Holden, J.M. & Sagousky, R. (1987) Detection of postnatal depression: development of the Edinburgh Postnatal Depression Scale. *British Journal of Psychiatry.* 130, 782–788.

Littlewood, J. & McHugh, N. (1997) *Maternal Distress and Postnatal Depression: The Myth of Madonna.* Basingstoke: Macmillan.

McIntosh, J. (1993) Postpartum depression: women's help-seeking behaviour and perceptions of cause. *Journal of Advanced Nursing.* 18:2, 178–184.

Elderly people

Duffy, D. (1997) Suicide in later life: how to spot risk factors. *Nursing Times.* 93:11, 56–57.

Lindesay, J. (1991) Suicide in the elderly. *International Journal of Geriatric Psychiatry.* 6:6, 355–361.

General

Williams, R. & Morgan, G. (eds) (1994) *Suicide Prevention: The Challenge Confronted.* London: HMSO.

8 RISK MANAGEMENT OF MENTALLY DISORDERED OFFENDERS IN THE COMMUNITY

Peter Wright and Ann Stockford

INTRODUCTION

This chapter is concerned with the risk assessment and management of mentally disordered offenders in the community and is divided into a number of sections. First, it refers to the policy and legislative framework; second, it describes the client group; and third, it outlines the relationship between mental disorder and violence. Fourth, the chapter then defines risk; fifth, it addresses risk assessment; and finally it considers issues of risk management.

Throughout the chapter the term 'practitioner' is used. This is a generic term which can apply to a number of professional disciplines including mental health nurses, but also social workers and probation officers, employed as front-line workers in community mental health settings. The term does not intend to devalue the specific skills or mandate of any particular professional group but does reflect the common professional issues, when engaged in such work. Where issues relating specifically to mental health nurses are addressed, this is made explicit.

The theme of the chapter is very broad. In order to make it more manageable, we concentrate on those people who have committed serious violent offences related to their mental disorder and who may present significant risk of reoffending. These service users are sometimes referred to as high-risk offenders. It is recognized that self-harm is more prevalent amongst mentally disordered offenders than violence to others. Therefore, readers seeking a review of self-harm issues are directed to Chapter 7.

The concept of community care for mentally disordered offenders is relatively new. Historically, provision has focused on custodial care and lagged behind other innovations in community mental health work. However, the last decade has witnessed increased interest in developing community-based services for this client group. Various reports and inquiries on prison suicides, the high rate of mental disorder among prisoners, the failings of the prison health care system and the treatment of patients in special hospitals (Hudson *et al.*, 1993) have raised the profile of offenders and have led to significant change in the organization and delivery of services. Mentally disordered offenders can no longer be considered 'the marginalized disenfranchised group they were in the recent past' (Stone, 1995, p.14). They 'have emerged from relative institutional obscurity to attain a much higher profile in the community' (Vaughan & Badger, 1995, p.*x*) and within criminal justice, health and social care agencies.

As mental health provision for offenders becomes more community based, it does so against a background of growing concern about the perceived risk of violence posed to the general public by mentally disordered people. Public anxiety has been fuelled by a number of highly publicized homicides where the inquiry reports (Blom-Cooper *et al.*, 1995; Dick *et al.*, 1991; Heginbotham *et al.*, 1994; Ritchie *et al.*, 1994; also see Sheppard, 1995) have found significant failings in the community management of mentally disordered offenders. Such failings create fear and anxiety in communities and undermine support for community care provision. Inquiries have repeatedly identified shortfalls in risk assessment and risk management procedures and focused attention on the current state of risk practice and the community supervision of mentally disordered people. Reed (1997) suggests that 'There is a need for better understanding of the relationship between mental disorder and risk and about what is involved in risk assessment and risk management' (p.4). This is now a central issue for health, social care and criminal justice agencies.

Accurate risk assessment and robust risk management are essential if nurses and other practitioners are to predict dangerous behaviours and be able to intervene appropriately to support high-risk service users safely in community settings. Public protection has to be a priority. In pursuance of this, agencies need to ensure that they have coherent ways of calculating risk, informed risk management strategies, risk audit and 'The ability to learn from best practice as well as from serious incident failures' (Kemshall, 1996, p.*viii*).

GOVERNMENT POLICY AND LEGISLATION

It is important for practitioners to understand the policy and legislative framework which informs good practice. This requires a knowledge of mental health and criminal justice domains. The move towards community care provision for mentally disordered offenders has been led by legislation, policy and procedural directives from the Home Office and /or Department of Health. Some are specific to mentally disordered offenders, (for example, Home Office Circular 66/90, 1990) but much is applicable to other offenders or people with mental health problems in general. There is now a large amount of policy and legislation, which in part is targeted at individuals considered to be potentially dangerous. The main thrust of such measures is focused on improved care management, close monitoring and supervision. This is to be achieved through the Care Programme Approach (CPA), supervision registers (National Health Service Management Executive [NHSME], 1994a) and supervised discharge orders (Mental Health Patients in the Community Act, 1995). These initiatives, when combined with the plethora of guidance on community care, provide a substantial framework for practice.

Of particular importance in relation to work with mentally disordered offenders was the Reed Report (Department of Health [DoH], 1992) which established the guiding principles that now underpin forensic mental health work. These are that care should be founded on regard for the quality of care and individual need, wherever possible provided in the community, under the least restrictive justifiable conditions and provided with the aim of maximizing rehabilitation and sustaining an independent life.

CLIENT GROUP

Mentally disordered offenders who have committed serious acts of violence (against people or property) may continue to be potentially dangerous in certain circumstances. Dangerousness is defined as posing a significant risk of physical or lasting psychological harm (HM Inspectorate of Probation, 1995). Offending may comprise offences such as homicide, attempted homicide, grievous bodily harm with intent, serious sexual offences, hostage taking, firearms offences, aggravated burglary or arson. These high-risk people present a potent image for the public and media (Carson, 1997), especially since they have already demonstrated their propensity for serious offending in the past. However, this needs to be kept in perspective since discharged forensic service users are more likely to relapse and require readmission than to reoffend or engage in violence even when isolated and poorly compliant with treatment (Lamb et al., 1988).

This group of service users are likely to have multiple needs and vulnerabilities, a long history of contact with a range of services and to be resource intensive. They may have severe mental illness, personality disorder or learning disabilities (and often dual or triple diagnosis). Many may lack insight into their mental disorder and have received treatment in coercive circumstances. It is worth noting that service users who present a risk to others are prone to vulnerability themselves and may be at risk of suicide, self-harm, self-neglect and exploitation.

MENTAL DISORDER AND RISK OF VIOLENCE

The connection between violent behaviour and serious mental disorder has been subject to media exaggeration and prejudice but a relationship does exist. Hollin & Howells (1993) suggest a consistent relationship between violence and the presence of mental disorder. It is important to emphasize that the elevated risk of violent offending is modest and that the vast majority of mentally disordered people do not commit offences and are no more dangerous than members of the general population. However, a number of factors have been identified that help define whether, and in what circumstances, mentally disordered people may behave in a dangerous way (Reed, 1997). These include a past history of violence, impulsivity, agitation and excitement, interpersonal sensitivity, high levels of anger/suspiciousness/hostility, clinical diagnosis (especially schizophrenia and personality/psychopathic disorder), active psychotic symptoms (such as delusions, command hallucinations and paranoid ideation), poor response to or non-compliance with prescribed medication, failure to maintain contact with support services and substance misuse (Alberg et al., 1996; McNeil & Binder, 1994; Steadman et al., 1993). Swanson and colleagues (1990) also found that multiple psychiatric diagnoses significantly increased the risk of violence. These factors appear to be cumulative. For example, a service user will present a greater risk to other people if they have a psychopathic disorder with active psychotic symptoms and concurrently misuse alcohol or drugs (Reed, 1997).

RISK DEFINED

Snowdon (1997) suggests that risk can be defined as the likelihood of an event occurring. While that event might be positive or negative, the concept of risk in mental disorder is more usually understood in terms of potential negative outcomes. Risk is multifaceted, dynamic and contextual. Some risks are general while others are more specific. 'It can be vigorously assessed, managed and reviewed' (Royal College of Psychiatrists [RCP], 1996, p.1) and although good practice can help reduce risk, it cannot be eliminated.

RISK ASSESSMENT

O'Rourke (1997a) defined risk assessment as a 'systematic collection of information to determine the degree to which the identified risk is present, or likely to pose problems at some point in the future' (p.104). It represents an informed judgement that requires a skilful consideration of a wide variety of risk factors, the significance of which will vary with individuals as their circumstances change.

As regards mental disorder, there are two methods of risk assessment: clinical and actuarial. Davison (1997) defines these terms thus.

> *Clinical assessment is that which occurs when information about risk factors is collated and interpreted through personal judgement, while actuarial assessment rests solely on empirically established relationships between data and the condition or event of interest.*

(p.201)

Clinical assessment aims to be a balanced judgement and informed opinion that seeks to explain and understand risk behaviour. It is based on interviewing, observation and reviewing service users' social history, looking at previous clinical notes and considering the results of psychological or neurological testing, if available. However, the method is subjective and dependent on the past experience, attitude and theoretical perspective of the assessor(s) and the quality of their relationship and interaction with the individual. It is also affected by the degree of service user compliance and their willingness to disclose information, as well as being prone to practitioner bias and value judgement.

Actuarial assessment is based on statistics and population studies. Measurements of risk are based on calculations of probability and by 'basing prediction of behaviour on the behaviour of others in similar circumstances' (Kemshall, 1996, p.10). It tends to produce general results rather than be person specific and is seen by some critics as static and mechanistic. The *Violence Prediction Scheme* (Webster *et al.*, 1994) and also *HCR20* (Webster *et al.*, 1995) are two of the best-known actuarial methods of assessing risk and dangerousness.

In terms of prediction, clinical assessment of risk has a poor record of accuracy, particularly of the risk of violence (Monahan, 1981). While actuarial assessment is claimed to fare a little better, it seems that the validity of both methods is only modestly greater than chance (Steadman, 1996). Prediction of recidivism is difficult. Statistical studies of risk assessment suggest that the prediction of violence indicates high rates of errors, usually in the area of overprediction (Steadman *et al.*, 1993). The accuracies of short-term predictions of violence have been found to be marginally better, although they are still overpredicted. Risk assessment in forensic mental health is thus an imperfect technology and at best a good guess. It is universally acknowledged as an imprecise science and a 'difficult skill of uncertain validity' (Reed, 1997).

Despite this, good practice and legal requirements dictate that practitioners working with offenders have to assess risk and dangerousness on a regular basis. In doing so, it is important that decision making is as accurate as possible in the light of current knowledge. It is clearly an injustice and affront to individual liberty to detain a person longer than necessary in conditions of security greater than their clinical needs merit. However, it is important that public safety is not compromised. Also, poor risk assessment, if shown to result in a service user reoffending, may end in litigation and agencies and practitioners need to understand the tort of negligence and their subsequent duty of care (Carson, 1996). Fortunately, there are encouraging developments to enhance the accuracy of risk assessment which need to be supported. While practice must acknowledge the limits of prediction, it needs to capitalize on the knowledge and expertise to date and provide clinically defensible decisions on the probability of violence. A number of authors have argued that combining clinical and actuarial methods represents best current practice and can improve the predictive ability of risk assessment (Carson, 1997; Jones, 1995; Monahan, 1997; RCP, 1996; Ryan, 1996).

Risk decisions, then, should be based on empirical evidence and clinical experience with actuarial approaches advocated as adjuncts to clinical judgement. Harris & Rice (1997) refer to this integrated approach as structuring discretion, using actuarial measures as an anchorpoint for clinical decision making. Webster and colleagues (1994), who have a distrust for unbridled clinical opinion, would support such an approach although caution needs to be exercised in the degree of any clinical override.

Whichever method of risk assessment is employed, risk factors will be central to the assessment process. As stated earlier, a number of risk factors have been consistently identified with violence and mental disorder. Thus, practitioners can feel confident knowing which factors are important, although the research literature has not demonstrated how these factors interact or which ones are as most influential. Such factors, referred to by Monahan & Steadman (1994) as 'theoretically coherent indices of risk' (p.*vii*), influence the likelihood of risk becoming manifest. Best practice suggests consideration of a range of factors covering demographics, psychiatric symptoms, personal proclivities and situational variants (Allen, 1997). There should also be reference to the impact of social issues, such as discrimination, stigma, isolation and poverty (Ryan, 1996). This is supported by Taylor (1985), who warns against ignoring the social, environmental and organic antecedents to mental disorder and violence. Significantly, Harris &

Rice (1997) and Crighton (1995) suggest that the most reliable factors that predict violence among mentally disordered offenders are the same as those that predict violence in offenders without mental health difficulties. Such characteristics pertain to antisocial personality, criminal or violent history, gender, age, marital status, social class and association with antisocial or criminal peers.

In relation to violence, a competent risk assessment will identify relevant factors involved in past behaviour, indicate the circumstances which may influence the service user's tendency to violence in the future (triggers) and estimate the likelihood of these recurring.

The aim is to assess the factors which have led the service user to be aggressive, to ascertain how many of those factors are amenable to change and then to intervene to alter the factors so that risks of aggression are reduced.

(Gunn, 1993, p.663).

The reduction of risk is therefore dependent on modifying risk factors for the individual service user and this should be addressed in the risk management strategy.

Risk assessment is an interactive process involving a sequence of decisions monitored and modified over a period of time. Government guidance HSG (94)27 (NHSME, 1994b) recommends a framework for assessing risk prior to a person's discharge from hospital and while placed in the community. Mental health nurses and other practitioners need to be familiar with its content. Good assessments are comprehensive and use data from a variety of sources. They may include reviewing third-party information (such as previous mental health and psychological reports, criminal records, police reports and victim statements), direct behavioural observation, clinical interview and psychometric testing (O'Rourke, 1997b). This view is supported by Potts (1995) who, in advocating the Home Office perspective, stressed that reasonable practice in risk assessment should display quality and range of information, as well as completeness and objectivity of analysis, concrete evidence of progress and realistic forward planning. Caution should be exercised in relation to the accuracy of service user self-report since this will depend on individual motivation and the anticipated consequences of disclosure. Some people will be less than truthful and deny or minimize their offending history.

Comprehensive assessments will be balanced and soundly argued. Assessments should have a multidisciplinary input and be client centred. They should seek carers' views (or those of significant others), be integral to the CPA and care management process and closely linked to the assessment of need. Assessments should also identify the person's strengths and indicate the resources required to manage risk effectively. Kemshall (1996) asserts that 'The use of combined clinical and actuarial assessment within such a dynamic and holistic framework is the most productive way forward for risk policy and practice guidance'. This supports the approach recommended by Hampshire Probation Service in their report *Recognising and Reducing Risk* (1995) and also O'Rourke (1997a) in developing *Risk Assessment Management and Audit System (RAMAS)*. RAMAS is a standardized scheme for measuring, monitoring and managing risk and can be employed by a range of practitioners including mental health nurses.

It is hoped that the development of such generic tools will enhance risk decisions although on a cautionary note, it is worth recollecting Prins (1996) who warns against the overzealous application of particular assessment models and is keen to dismiss the idea that there is a highly sophisticated approach to the basics of risk assessment. It is also sobering to recollect Scott (1977) who states that it is 'patience, thoroughness and persistence in the process of information gathering rather than any diagnostic brilliance' (p.129) that provides the surest approach to the assessment of risk.

RISK MANAGEMENT ISSUES

Risk management is the process of planning and decision making for individual offenders and the development of strategies (medical, psychological and social) to reduce the severity and frequency of identified adverse risks. It aims to help structure thinking, increase the likelihood of quality risk decisions and positive risk outcomes. It is described by Carson (1990) as an ongoing and directed programme with regular proactive reviews to enable more strategic, informed and defensible decisions to be made. Risk management needs to be based on a clear policy, established protocol, prescribed procedures and best practice guidelines. Having identified risk, there is an absolute duty of care to manage it. The consequences of agencies failing to provide adequate care and control for high-risk offenders are potentially catastrophic. Public and staff safety would be compromised, as would the clinical reputation of services and individual practitioners. Risk management systems should enable consistent, reliable and credible decision making which should be justifiable with hindsight in circumstances of serious reoffending.

Agencies and individual practitioners are, of course, accountable for the quality of their practice if not always for the outcome of their risk decisions (although this is invariably linked). Risk is inherent in mental health work and services cannot be provided on a no-risk basis. A balance needs to be struck between risk minimization and risk taking which empowers service users and leads to greater independence (Ryan, 1993). Inevitably, some decisions will have negative outcomes. However, providing reasonable practice has been adhered to and clear guidelines on risk assessment and management exist, this may need to be an acceptable, though regrettable consequence of a progressive health and social care policy.

Controls in the community

Most high-risk offenders are likely to be subject to statutory coercive controls in the community. A number of measures can be applied. Some people will be conditionally discharged from a hospital order but still subject to Home Office restrictions. Others will be on leave of absence, but still formally detained under the Mental Health Act (1983). Conditionally discharged service users are required to reside at a place approved by the Home Secretary and to accept mental health and social supervision. They may also have to comply with medication, avoid returning to the area of the index offence and could be prohibited from having contact with particular individuals such as victims or victims' relatives. If a service user does not comply with the requirements imposed, they may be recalled to hospital.

All people detained under the Mental Health Act (1983) will be subject to section 117 where health authorities and social services have a legal obligation to provide appropriate aftercare. Furthermore, service users will be subject to the CPA which requires a systematic assessment of health and social care needs, a key worker to co-ordinate care, a written care plan and regular review. Service users could also be liable to supervised discharge which applies to previously detained but non-restricted people and provides the framework to ensure compliance with aftercare arrangements. Failure to do so would lead to a review and possibly readmission to hospital. Service users who present a serious risk to themselves or others may also be on a supervision register. Practitioners may additionally work with people subject to guardianship orders (Mental Health Act, 1983) or probation orders with conditions for mental health treatment.

Practitioners will apply or help police such community controls and need to be aware of their legal responsibility and accountability in doing so. Community mental health nurses are one of the most likely disciplines to act as the CPA key worker for service users not subject to Home Office restrictions. This may involve an obligation to ensure that risk is assessed, communicated and managed. There is concern within the nursing profession about potential legal repercussions, as well as the increased social control role being asked of nurses (Allen, 1997).

Preparation for discharge

Effective management of the transition from inpatient to community care is crucial. Transition is a potentially high-risk time and a gradual staged process of rehabilitation will help minimize risk. People with histories of serious offending and mental disorder will have been subject to prolonged periods of hospitalization. Discharge from hospital will need to be planned with a gradual reduction in the level of security and restrictions on individuals. Service users will normally follow a programme of escorted and unescorted periods of parole, first within the hospital grounds and then further afield within the local area. There should be day visits, overnight and weekend home leaves or leaves to the supervised residential accommodation to which service users will be discharged. There is a need for careful preparation and adequate links between hospital and those nurses and other practitioners who are to supervise the offender in the community.

Ideally, a continuum of care needs to be maintained. This should be provided by a clinical team with responsibility for care during hospitalization, transition and in the community for those people who continue to live locally. The community mental health nurse and social worker who are to be responsible for aftercare once the service user is discharged need to be involved at an early stage in order for relationships with the user to be developed and future care and treatment planned. This is in line with CPA and such practitioners are in a key position to assess the home or residential accommodation and provide support for carers and aftercare agencies.

Moving from the regimented institutional setting of a secure unit, which provides a large measure of physical security, to a less structured setting based more on relational security and high supervision presents a degree of anxiety for service providers and users alike. As noted by Jones (1995) citing Bailey & MacCulloch (1992):

> Careful observation is required on how service users adjust to a new environment and how they cope with increased personal responsibility and freedom. This period can be very unsettling and when under stress, clients could relapse, or return to old, potentially dangerous patterns of behaviour.
>
> (p.10).

Individuals may also act out to consciously or unconsciously seek reassurance that the new support system is capable of responding and setting limits (Kaliski, 1997).

Community supervision

The community supervision of potentially dangerous people necessitates a higher degree of surveillance than is usual in traditional mental health work. There is a need to adopt a more assertive approach that is 'well planned, purposeful and at times necessarily determined' (HM Inspectorate of Probation, 1995, p.9). The monitoring nature of the relationship needs to be acknowledged and a balance attained between care and control: between a service user's rights and welfare and the rights of the public to be protected from avoidable harm. In clinical practice, this should not present a conflict of interest since freedom from appropriate supervision only to kill or seriously harm again is not in the service user's interest (Taylor, 1997).

Close monitoring and intensive care management while under community supervision provide opportunities for ongoing and frequent assessments of a person's mental health, their compliance with treatment and potential difficulties. Such supervision permits prompt action when the likelihood of serious risk becomes evident. It can also test progress and instil confidence. Bates (1995) indicated that regular high-quality contact between forensic community nurses and their service users can reduce the likelihood of dangerousness and Bloom & Williams (1994) showed that contact maintained with mental health practitioners over a prolonged period is associated with positive outcomes. Practitioners need to be pragmatically cautious, constantly vigilant and observant and have a good eye for detail. They should be thorough and persistent with a sensitivity to the risk of the service user reoffending and history repeating itself (Vaughan & Badger, 1995). An ability to pick up on cues about behaviour is important. A degree of healthy scepticism should be maintained, tempering practitioners' natural optimism about a service user's capacity to change. Prins (1990) stresses the need to develop a high threshold of suspiciousness and a capacity to ask the unimaginable, unthinkable and unaskable questions.

Risk issues need to be regularly raised and monitored and, where appropriate, behaviour and attitudes challenged. Practice should emphasize public protection and practitioners need to act in the public interest if an offender's behaviour is likely to pose a threat to public safety. There is a need for regular contact with service users, careful monitoring and swift action when necessary to forestall dangerous behaviour. Good record keeping and a high standard of documentation are important, in terms of not only communication but also accountability. The importance of accurate and precise recording of information cannot be overestimated.

In working with high-risk offenders, the establishment of a constructive therapeutic relationship with the service user is important. Great value is placed on long-term supervision by practitioners who know the person well in order to provide a degree of continuity. Continuity correlates positively with successful reintegration and safe community management (Norris, 1984). It is equally important to enlist the support of the service user in helping monitor their own well-being for, without their co-operation and agreement, management of risk will be more difficult. It should be noted that it takes time to develop trust and service users may only reveal things when a good rapport has been established. Care should be provided by a multidisciplinary team that knows the person well. The team should have a stable membership and a commitment to long-term involvement with the user. Care management is likely to be intensive and service users require high-quality, close supervision and contact with mental health services, even when they are mentally well. Postdischarge supervision may need to continue indefinitely for some people. Lengthy periods of supervision are associated with lower rates of recidivism.

Interagency working

The needs of high-risk offenders are complex and cannot be met by a single agency or any one profession. 'The safe management of previously violent offenders in the community thus requires careful, well organized and well resourced services working in collaboration and partnership with each other' (Chiswick, 1995, p.236). The Reed Report (DoH, 1992) emphasized the importance of interagency working at strategic, operational and care management levels and a well-integrated seamless range of services should be the aim of planners and service managers. However, the demands on time and resource costs of good joint working should be acknowledged in the planning and costing of services. There should be strong connections between key agencies involved in the person's care. There also need to be appropriate multidisciplinary and interagency meetings in order to discuss individual client and practice issues. Such meetings can offer support and advice and enhance communication and decision making. In terms of liaison, community mental health nurses can make a core contribution through acting as the central contact with the service user and the various agencies involved in their care.

It is also important for agencies to be aware of their own limitations and for practitioners not to work beyond their level of competence, as highlighted in the inquiry into the death of Jonathan Newby (Davies et al., 1995). A supportive approach should be developed which fosters a culture of agencies being able to call on one another's expertise, knowledge, resources and, where appropriate, statutory powers. Joint policies, procedures and strategies need to be agreed between agencies in managing situations of risk, if interagency work is to be effective; for example, in the sharing of relevant information about individual service users. Failure to pass on information can put service users, practitioners and others at risk. This is illustrated in the *Report of the Inquiry into the Care and Treatment of Christopher Clunis* (Ritchie *et al.*, 1994) which criticized agencies for failing to communicate, share information and liaise effectively.

Interagency protocol for information sharing should be established. The Department of Health (1996a) has produced guidance on the protection and use of service user information within the NHS and it would be good practice if other agencies involved with mentally disordered offenders considered the need for similar guidance. *Building Bridges* (DoH, 1996b) is useful in this respect. Agencies should have written policies with mechanisms for disclosing information which should be available for service users to inspect. It needs to be stressed that because of the coercive context in which community supervision is generally delivered, practitioners 'need to be especially sensitive to the issues of confidentiality and diligent in explaining its absence or limitations to clients' (Hollin & Howells, 1993, p.226). Central to good practice with high-risk offenders is the fact that interests of public protection should take precedence over the right to confidentiality.

Multidisciplinary teamwork

A consistent, comprehensive and multidisciplinary approach should be adopted which advocates networking, good communication and information sharing between disciplines. Such teamwork made up of mental health nurses, psychiatrists, psychologists, social workers and occupational therapists, is of vital importance in the community supervision of high-risk service users. It can enrich practice and provide opportunities for joint work, sharing of tasks and mutual support. An effective team is always greater than the sum of its individual parts. It allows practitioners to draw on a range of different skills and enables more creative practice. Multidisciplinary teamwork, though, can be challenging since professionals come from different disciplines, will have received different training, have different conditions of employment and differences in perceived status and prestige (Prins, 1983). Good working relationships with colleagues require a degree of openness, trust and respect for one another's contributions. A degree of flexibility among practitioners and some blurring of professional boundaries is also necessary. However, a particular problem to be avoided in multidisciplinary work is the failure to assign clear lines of responsibility and accountability.

Services

There are two main approaches to supporting high-risk offenders in the community: supervised residential provision and assertive outreach support. These services can be provided by a forensic team or generic mental health practitioners working in close collaboration with forensic services. In terms of accommodation, some people will need high levels of support and supervision and require access to 24-hour nursed care. Others can be supported in self-contained accommodation close to a 24-hour staffed residential unit (along the lines of a core and cluster model). Assertive outreach, on the other hand, provides support to individuals living in independent accommodation. It can be described as intensive care management based on intervention being initiated by the agency or practitioner, rather than the service user. The outreach team need a degree of flexibility in responding to service user need and should be able to visit regularly during the day, evenings and weekends. Some form of out-of-hours crisis support will be necessary.

Examples of high supervision accommodation and assertive outreach include Turning Point's Alfred Minto House (AMH) in Nottingham and the Gwydir Project in Cambridge. AMH is a specialist residential unit providing accommodation, resettlement and social care for people who have previously been detained in secure environments. The focus of its work is on risk management and the prevention of reoffending. Such units are neither cheap nor easy to run and the Social Service Inspectorate (DoH, 1996c), while advocating the need for such facilities, acknowledged the shortage of such accommodation. The Gwydir Project provides intensive outreach support to people deemed to present significant risk to themselves or others. It functions through interagency co-operation, providing continuous flexible care in line with the type of services advocated in the report of Ritchie *et al.* (1994).

The Home Office guidelines on social supervision (Home Office/Department of Health & Social Security, 1987) state that public protection is best assured by effective management and successful integration of mentally disordered offenders into the community. Practitioners should therefore have a positive and constructive approach to community supervision, rather than simply monitoring progress. As part of managing risk, there are a number of therapeutic interventions which can be employed (many of which are discussed in other chapters of this volume), such as emphasis on medication, anger or anxiety management, treatment of alcohol or substance abuse, offence-focused work and problem-solving skills. Community supervision should also be characterized by a large measure of practical support. Service elements need to include proactive intervention to access appropriate accommodation, intervention to ensure full take-up of Benefit Agency entitlements, the use of occupation, education and social opportunities and enhancement of a service user's family and social relationships.

Crises

Circumstances which give cause for concern are when there appears to be an actual or potential increase in risk, contact with the service user is lost or they are unwilling to co-operate with aftercare arrangements (Home Office/DHSS, 1987). If a person's behaviour or mental health deteriorates, this may necessitate further inpatient treatment. Careful monitoring is essential so that the potential threat of dangerous behaviour can be quickly identified (Lawrie, 1997). Early identification of warning signs is important in order to intervene and prevent relapse or recidivism. The aim is to avoid deterioration of the service user to a point of presenting a danger to themselves or others or reoffending and having to be arrested or readmitted to hospital in traumatic and possibly dramatic circumstances (Vaughan & Badger, 1995). In order to support a person in crisis within the community, a capacity for rapid response is required and there needs to be access to on-call, 24-hour support from a community mental health nurse and social worker who have back-up from either a duty doctor or consultant.

Crisis management may employ a combination of therapeutic and controlling interventions. The use of calming and defusing methods to reduce emotional arousal and negotiation and medication to reduce conflict may also be advised (Harris & Rice, 1997). Concerns should be addressed by the multidisciplinary team and the management and treatment plan reviewed. If a service user presents significant risk, admission to hospital, informally or under civil section, will be required. For a restricted conditionally discharged service user, recall to hospital may be appropriate, although informal admission may suffice to stabilize them without recourse to recall proceedings. If recalled, there is a specific set procedure to follow and the person will need to be informed of the reasons for recall and their rights under the Mental Health Act (1983).

Safety

Personal safety is an issue in working with high-risk service users. Agencies must accept the responsibility for providing practitioners with a working environment that is personally safe and with the interagency resources for appropriate back-up, continuing care and crisis support. Work places need to be safe without being oppressive. Basic precautions might include 'toughened glass screens for receptionists, coded locks and viewing panels to doors and duress alarms (panic buttons) within individual offices' (HM Inspectorate of Probation, 1995, p.67). Controlled access to buildings is recommended.

In addition, adherence to safe working practice is necessary. This may include having staff check on colleagues (either by phone or in person) who may be meeting on site with a potentially violent service user and being informed where and how long meetings are to last. If practitioners are working outside agency premises then a system of checking in and out with office staff before and after meetings with individual service users is required. Procedures also need to be in place for informing the police if practitioners fail to report in. Practitioners may also need a mobile phone and they should visit in pairs if particularly concerned about a person or a potentially difficult situation. They should also be aware of good practice in managing a potential, or actual, violent situation which needs to be supported by mandatory practical training. It is crucial to recognize that safety depends at least as much on the confidence, skills and attitudes of the practitioners (relational security) as it does on procedures and physical security.

Staff support

Professional involvement in risk management with the high-risk offender can be a demanding task; the complexity of the work, the nature of some index offences, the risk of violence and the potential for disaster if things go wrong present considerable challenge (Vaughan & Badger, 1995). For many practitioners there will be periods of high anxiety, ambiguity, uncertainty and vulnerability. Drawing on Prins (1986), Vaughan & Badger (1995) cite that 'There is little doubt that some offenders can fill practitioners with an intangible disquiet and even apprehension' (p.168). Work with high-risk and possible high-profile service users in community settings is stressful and good systems of support are necessary if practitioners are to have an empowering foundation for practice. Practitioners need to be competent, well supervised and appropriately trained. High-risk offenders should not have junior staff as key workers unless tightly managed by experienced supervisors and then not for long periods. In forensic services, it is important to acknowledge the need for practitioners to have reduced or protected caseloads and for working environments to have high staff service : user ratios.

In general, practitioners need to feel supported by line management who should have working knowledge of individual high-risk service users and active involvement in key risk management decisions. This is important, in terms not only of support but also accountability. Lawrie (1997) suggests first-line managers need to be 'knowledgeable and experienced in order to advise, endorse or guide interventions and to coach practitioners in order to enhance professional skills' (p.303). Managers will need to check that risk assessments are appropriate and risk management strategies adhered to.

Practitioners should be given the opportunity to explore their own feelings and regular individual clinical supervision is essential. It is important to ensure that 'distress, collusion, error and bias within practitioners are constructively dealt with and that effective intervention strategies are pursued' (Kemshall, 1996, p.33). Supervision of individual workers should be further enhanced through staff appraisal and linked to training opportunities. Beacock (1994) demonstrated the value of staff development for forensic nurses in maintaining commitment, staff moral and increased job satisfaction. In addition to individual supervision, group supervision with an independent and experienced supervisor, as described by Stanley (1996), or a staff support group with interagency membership can also be useful. There is great value in formal and informal support from colleagues and other professionals involved in the risk management process. Also, access to additional support and debriefing should be available after distressing incidents or negative outcomes. Staff support can also be enhanced by good leadership, clear aims and objectives, good working environments and terms and conditions of employment and sufficient funding.

Training

Best practice will require knowledgeable, competent and skilled staff with specialized knowledge and expertise. Practitioners working with high-risk offenders should be experienced and confident. Training should recognize that the analysis of risk and the development of decision-making skills is important at basic and postqualifying levels. There is a place for both internal and interagency training and comprehensive training materials on risk are available, for example

Learning Materials on Risk Assessment (Alberg *et al.*, 1996) which was commissioned by the Department of Health and Social Service Inspectorate. Snowdon (1997) asserts that risk assessment and management is more of an approach than a skill and difficult to teach in a classroom situation isolated from care environments. Snowdon believes training is best provided in an apprenticeship situation, within a forensic placement, supplemented by specific teaching sessions.

The role of continuing professional education on a multidisciplinary basis involving other community staff is important. Kemshall (1996) highlights that training will need to consider the complex nature of risk and issues involved in risk prediction. It needs to identify appropriate texts and the factors most appropriate for assessment of risk in mental health (Harris, 1997). It should also address both clinical and actuarial methods of risk assessment, their strengths and deficits and how they can be combined to be more effective. Training should provide the necessary skills and techniques for risk assessment models to be applied properly, to inform practitioners of risk management strategies and to stress the importance of monitoring and reviewing risk.

CONCLUSION

The task of assessment and community management of risk is often 'complex, emotional and morally challenging' (Carson, 1990, p.60). Such work is at the early stage of development although in recent years the knowledge base has increased significantly. There is now sufficient evidence from research, clinical practice and inquiry reports to demonstrate the practice required to reduce serious and unnecessary risks. However, good risk practice will be frustrated if the managerial support, resources and staff training are not available to enable it to be realized. This is one of the challenges for mental health services as we enter the new millennium.

REFERENCES

Alberg, C., Hatfield, B. & Huxley, P. (1996) *Learning Materials on Mental Health Risk Assessment*. Manchester: Manchester University and Department of Health.

Allen, J. (1997) Assessing and managing risk of violence in the mentally disordered. *Journal of Psychiatric and Mental Health Nursing*. 4:5, 369–378.

Bailey, J. & MacCulloch, M. (1992) Patterns of reconviction in patients discharged directly to the community from a special hospital: implications for aftercare. *Journal of Forensic Psychiatry*. 3:3, 445–461.

Bates, A. (1995) Mental disorder and criminal behaviour. *Psychiatric Care*. 2:3, 96–100.

Beacock, C. (1994) Journey without end: creating a development strategy for staff in secure provision. In: T. Thompson & P. Mathias (eds) *Lyttle's Mental Health and Disorder*, 2nd edn. London: Baillière Tindall, pp. 535–551.

Blom-Cooper, L., Hally, H. & Murphy, E. (1995) *The Falling Shadow: One Patient's Mental Health Care 1978–93*. London: Duckworth.

Bloom, J. & Williams, M. (1994) *Management and Treatment of Insanity Acquitees: A Model for the 1990's*. Washington, DC: American Psychiatric Press.

Carson, D. (ed) (1990) *Risk-taking in Mental Disorder: Analyses, Policies and Practical Strategies*. Chichester: SLE Publications.

Carson, D. (1996) Risking legal repercussions. In: H. Kemshall & J. Pritchard (eds) *Good Practice in Risk Assessment and Risk Management*, Volume 1. London: Jessica Kingsley Publications, pp. 3–13.

Carson, D. (1997) Good enough risk taking. *International Review of Psychiatry*. 9, 303–308.

Chiswick, D. (1995) Dangerousness. In: D. Chiswick & R. Cope (eds) *Seminars in Practical Forensic Psychiatry*. London: Royal College of Psychiatrists/Gaskell, pp. 210–240.

Crighton, J. (ed) (1995) *Psychiatric Patient Violence: Risk and Response*. London: Duckworth.

Davies, N., Lingham, R., Prior, C. & Sims, A. (1995) *Report of the Inquiry into the Circumstances Leading to the Death of Jonathan Newby (a Volunteer Worker)*. Oxford: Oxfordshire Health Authority.

Davison, S. (1997) Risk assessment and management: a busy practitioner's perspective. *International Review of Psychiatry*. 9:2-3, 201–206.

Department of Health (1992) *Review of Health and Social Services for Mentally Disordered Offenders*. London: HMSO.

Department of Health (1996a) *The Protection and Use of Patient Information: Guidance from the Department of Health*. London: HMSO.

Department of Health (1996b) *Building Bridges: A Guide to Arrangements for Interagency Working for the Care and Protection of Severely Mentally Ill People*. London: HMSO.

Department of Health (1996c) *Improving Services for Mentally Disordered Offenders*. London: Social Services Inspectorate/HMSO.

Dick, D., Shuttleworth, B. & Carlton, J. (1991) *Report of the Panel of Inquiry Appointed by the West Midlands Regional Health Authority and Special Hospitals Service Authority to Investigate the Case of Kim Kirkham*. Birmingham: West Midlands Regional Health Authority.

Gunn, J. (1993) Dangerousness. In: J. Gunn & P. Taylor (eds) *Forensic Psychiatry: Clinical, Legal and Ethical Issues*. Oxford: Butterworth Heinemann, pp. 624–645.

Hampshire Probation Service (1995) *Recognising and Reducing Risk. Improving the Quality of Decisions in Situations which Threaten Harm. An Interim Report of the Risk Management Working Party*. Southampton: Hampshire Probation Service.

Harris, G. & Rice, M. (1997) Risk appraisal and management of violent behaviour. *Psychiatric Services*. 48: 9, 1168–1176.

Harris, M. (1997) Training trainers in risk assessment. *British Journal of Psychiatry*. 170 (supplement 32), 35–36.

Heginbotham, C., Carr, J., Hole, R., Walsh, T. & Warren, L. (1994) *Report of the Independent Panel of Inquiry Examining the Case of Michael Buchanan*. London: North West London NHS Trust.

HM Inspectorate of Probation (1995) *Dealing with Dangerous People: The Probation Service and Public Protection – Report of a Thematic Inspection*. London: Home Office.

Hollin, C. & Howells, K. (1993) *Clinical Approaches to the Mentally Disordered Offender*. Chichester: John Wiley.

Home Office (1990) *Provision for Mentally Disordered Offenders*. London: Home Office (Circular No. 66/90).

Home Office and Department of Health and Social Security (1987) *Mental Health Act 1983 Supervision and Aftercare of Conditionally Discharged Restricted Patients: Notes for the Guidance of Social Supervisors*. London: Home Office.

Hudson, B., Cullen, R. & Roberts, C. (1993) *Training for Work with Mentally Disordered Offenders*. London: Central Council for Education and Training in Social Work.

Jones, D. (1995) *Prediction of Dangerousness*. London: Special Hospital Services Authority. Unpublished paper.

Kaliski, Z. (1997) Risk management during the transition from hospital to community care. *International Review of Psychiatry*. 9:2–3, 249–256.

Kemshall, H. (1996) *Reviewing Risk – A Review of Research on the Assessment and Management of Risk and Dangerousness: Implications for Policy and Practice in the Probation Service*. A Report for the Home Office Research and Statistics Directorate. Croydon: Home Office.

Lamb, H., Weinberger, L. & Gross, B. (1988) Court mandated community out-patient treatment for persons found not guilty by reason of insanity: a five year follow up. *American Journal of Psychiatry*. 145, 450–456.

Lawrie, C. (1997) Risk: the role and responsibilities of middle managers. In: H. Kemshall & J. Pritchard (eds) *Good Practice in Risk Assessment and Risk Management*, Volume 2. London: Jessica Kingsley Publications, pp. 301–311.

McNeil, D. & Binder, R. (1994) The relationship between acute psychiatric symptoms, diagnosis and short term risk of violence. *Hospital and Community Psychiatry*. 45:2, 133–137.

Mental Health Act (1983) London: HMSO.

Mental Health (Patients in the Community) Act (1995) London: HMSO.

Monahan, J. (1981) *The Clinical Prediction of Violence*. Beverly Hills, California: Sage.

Monahan, J. (1997) Actuarial support for the clinical assessment of violence risk. *International Review of Psychiatry*. 9:2–3, 167–169.

Monahan, J. & Steadman, H. (eds) (1994) *Violence and Mental Disorder: Developments in Risk Assessment*. Chicago, Illinois: University of Chicago Press.

National Health Service Management Executive (1994a) *Introduction of Supervision Registers for Mentally Ill People from 1 April 1994*. London: HMSO (NSG (94)5).

National Health Service Management Executive (1994b) *Guidance on the Discharge of Mentally Disordered People and their Continuing Care in the Community*. London: HMSO (HSG (94) 27).

Norris, M. (1984) *Integration of Special Hospital Patients into the Community*. Aldershot: Gower.

O'Rourke, M. (1997a) Risk assessment and risk management: the way forward. *Psychiatric Care*. 4:3, 104–106.

O'Rourke, M. (1997b) Assessment and treatment of sex offenders. *Psychiatric Care*. 4:6, 258–264.

Potts, J. (1995) Risk assessment and management: a Home Office perspective. In: J. Crighton (ed) *Psychiatric Patient Violence: Risk and Response*. London: Duckworth, pp. 35–43.

Prins, H. (1983) The care of the psychiatric prisoner: discharge into the community and its implications. *Medical Science and the Law.* 23:2, 79–86.

Prins, H. (1986) *Dangerous Behaviour: The Law and Mental Disorder.* London: Tavistock.

Prins, H. (1990) The supervision of potentially dangerous offender patients in England and Wales. *International Journal of Offender Therapy and Comparative Criminology.* 34:3, 213–221.

Prins, H. (1996) Risk assessment and management in criminal justice and psychiatry. *Journal of Forensic Psychiatry.* 7:1, 42–62.

RCP (1996) *Assessment and Clinical Management of Risk of Harm to Other People.* London: Royal College of Psychiatrists (Report CR53).

Reed, J. (1997) Risk assessment and clinical management: the lessons from recent inquiries. *British Journal of Psychiatry.* 170 (Supplement 32), 4–7.

Ritchie, J., Dick, D. & Lingham, R. (1994) *The Report of the Inquiry into the Care and Treatment of Christopher Clunis.* London: HMSO.

Ryan, T. (1993) Therapeutic risks in mental health nursing. *Nursing Standard.* 7: 24, 29–31.

Ryan, T. (1996) Risk management and people with mental health problems. In: H. Kemshall & J. Pritchard (eds) *Good Practice in Risk Assessment and Risk Management,* Volume 1. London: Jessica Kingsley Publications, pp. 93–109.

Scott, P. (1977) Assessing dangerousness in criminals. *British Journal of Psychiatry.* 131, 127–142.

Sheppard, D. (1995) *Learning the Lessons: Mental Health Inquiry Reports Published in England and Wales between 1969 and 1996 and their Recommendations for Improving Practice.* London: Zito Trust.

Snowdon, P. (1997) Practical aspects of clinical assessment and management. *British Journal of Psychiatry.* 170 (Supplement 32), 32–34.

Stanley, A. (1996) The impact of the first forensic encounter: a trainee's view. In: C. Cordess & M. Cox (eds) *Forensic Psychotherapy: Crime, Psychodynamics and the Offender Patient,* Volume 2. London: Jessica Kingsley Publications, pp. 225–228.

Steadman, H. (1996) The MacArthur Violence Risk Assessment Study. Paper presented at the *Violence, Competence and Coercion: The Pivotal Issues in Mental Health Law Conference.* MacArthur Foundation Research Network on Mental Health and the Law. Oxford, 4–5 July.

Steadman, H., Monahan, J., Robbins, P. *et al.* (1993) From dangerousness to risk assessment: implications for appropriate research strategies. In: S. Hodgkins (eds) *Mental Disorder and Crime.* Beverly Hills, California: Sage, pp. 39–62.

Stone, N. (1995) *A Companion Guide to Mentally Disordered Offenders.* Ilkley: Owen Wells.

Swanson, J., Holzer, C., Ganju, V.K. & Jono, R. (1990) Violence and psychiatric disorder in the community: evidence from Epidemiological Catchment Area surveys. *Hospital and Community Psychiatry.* 41:7, 761–770.

Taylor, P. (1985) Motives for offending among violent and psychotic men. *British Journal of Psychiatry.* 147, 491–498.

Taylor, P. (1997) Mental disorder and risk of violence. *International Review of Psychiatry.* 9:2–3, 157–161.

Vaughan, P. & Badger, D. (1995) *Working with the Mentally Disordered Offender in the Community.* London: Chapman & Hall.

Webster, C., Harris, G., Rice, M., Cormier, C. & Bounds, V. (1994) *The Violence Prediction Scheme: Assessing Dangerousness in High Risk Men.* Toronto: Centre for Criminology, University of Toronto.

Webster, C. & Eaves, D. with Douglas, K. & Wintrop, A. (1995) *The HCR 20 Scheme. The Assessment of Dangerousness and Risk.* Vancouver: Simon Frazer University and Forensic Psychiatric Services Commission of British Columbia.

CRISIS INTERVENTION AND RISK MANAGEMENT
WITH SEX OFFENDERS

Pauline England, Maeve Murphy and Jim Duckworth

Sex offenders have become the new bogeymen, used by politicians to intimidate and scare citizens concerned about public safety. Often the claims have more to do with scoring political points than creating a safer society.

(Lotke, 1996, p.1)

INTRODUCTION

Of all the crimes which worry us, perhaps sexual offences are the most frightening, especially to parents who fear for the safety of their children. There are times when it seems impossible to open a newspaper without seeing another article about a sex offender. This doubtless reflects society's deep anxieties about a behaviour which has such serious consequences for its victims. Many people cannot comprehend such behaviour and most seem to prefer not to think about it if at all possible. For mental health nurses, this stance is incompatible with their professional responsibilities for many will encounter sex offenders in the course of their work. This chapter seeks to assist mental health nurses in managing the risks posed by this client group.

DEFINITIONS AND DEMOGRAPHY

In this chapter the term 'sex offender' is taken to apply to:

- someone who has committed an illegal sexual act with another person (such as indecent exposure, indecent assault, unlawful sexual intercourse, buggery or rape) and/or;
- someone whose behaviour, while not inherently illegal, undermines the victim's sexual safety or sexual identity (such as exposing children to pornography or engaging them in inappropriately explicit sexual conversations) (Vancouver Society for Male Survivors of Sexual Abuse, 1995).

How many people commit sexual offences? The most important thing to realize about sex offenders is that we do not know who most of them are (Lotke, 1996). According to the Home Office (Marshall, 1997), about one in 90 men born in 1953 had a conviction by the age of 40 for a serious sexual offence (e.g. rape, buggery, incest, unlawful sexual intercourse). When less serious offences are included, the figure is one in 40. The Home Office estimated that in 1993 at least

260,000 men aged 20 or over had been convicted of a sexual offence and of these, 110,000 were for offences against children (Marshall, 1997).

Although most sex offenders are men, women do also commit sexual offences. Finkelhor (1986) writes that in reported cases of child sexual abuse, 90% of offenders are men. Fisher (1994) reports that at any one time there are 3000 adult male sex offenders in prison and 12 female. Therefore, since the overwhelming majority of sexual offenders are men, it is upon them that this chapter will focus.

The range of people affected by sexual offences is very wide. A sexual offence can have a serious impact on many more people than the immediate victim. Their family and friends will have to come to terms with what has happened and there may be very difficult problems for a sexual partner to deal with. The family and friends of the offender also have to deal with the consequences of the offence(s). Indeed, they may be harassed themselves because of it.

When a local community discovers that a sexual offence has been committed in their area, many people feel very anxious. Women especially may be afraid to go out alone or parents will not allow their children to play outside. Many parents, perhaps particularly fathers, have become anxious about being naked around their children and concerned about cuddling them. Those who work with the victims/survivors or perpetrators of sexual offences also have to deal with their own emotional response to such devastating crimes.

Much of the therapeutic work in this field has been carried out by probation or prison officers. There has been relatively little interest from mental health professionals. Indeed, in some people's minds, being a nurse or doctor would be a positive disqualification because these professions are associated with ideas about *illness* and the *medical model* which are seen as counterproductive in this area of work. From the client's point of view, there are two possible disadvantages. Although it is difficult to imagine being more stigmatized than being called a sex offender or child molester, perhaps being labelled 'mad' is worse. On the other hand, the idea that a mental illness caused one to commit sexual offences may be a comforting thought for some people that insulates them from taking responsibility for the devastation they have caused in other people's lives.

The consensus of those working in this field is that while a few sex offenders have a serious mental illness, the vast majority do not. Instead, they have made a number of decisions and choices that have gradually culminated in their offending behaviour (Mander et al., 1996). The issue is also clouded by the use of the term 'treatment' to describe work that confronts sex offenders in order to change their offending behaviour. As the term is in common use, it is used within this chapter, but readers are asked to remember that it is the choices and decisions of clients with which we seek to work and so reduce the risk of the client offending again (Faulk, 1988). Indeed, there are those who believe that statistical studies alone produce more reliable estimates of risk than clinical assessments (Webster, 1995).

It probably comes as a surprise to most people that offenders, especially those who have been treated, are less likely to reoffend than other types of offenders.

Box 9.1

Recidivism rates of selected offenders

Type of offender	% re-offending
Treated sex offenders	10.9%
Untreated sex offenders	18.8%
Drug offenders	25.0%
Violent offenders	30.0%

(Adapted from Lotke, 1996)

RECIDIVISM

Sex offenders who have been caught and punished are probably less of a threat to society than other groups of offenders (Quinsey et al., 1995). Most sex offenders are never convicted of another sexual offence (Lotke, 1996). The typical sex offender appears in court once and then never again, at least for a further sex crime (Hanson & Bussière, 1996).

In addition, much research has shown that the risk of reoffending is higher where there is a greater number of previous offences and deviant sexual arousal (Grubin & Wingate, 1996). Quinsey and colleagues (1995) found that the degree of psychopathy shown by an offender was a reliable indicator of risk (Motiuk & Brown, 1996). There are differences in risk level which relate to the type of offence previously committed. Rapists tend to reoffend more often than offenders against children while, in respect to offences against children, incest offenders are least likely to reoffend (Hanson & Bussière, 1996; Motiuk & Brown, 1996; Quinsey et al., 1995). The next most risky sexual offenders are those who offended against unrelated female victims (Quinsey et al., 1995), while the offenders most likely to reoffend are those whose victims are boys (Motiuk & Brown, 1996; Quinsey et al., 1995). More positively, Grubin & Wingate (1996) found that being married and being employed acted as protection against reoffending (Hanson & Bussière, 1996; Quinsey et al., 1995).

RISK ASSESSMENT

In attempting to assess the risk posed by an offender, it is useful to think of risk as a continuum and to remember that the risk from an individual may change over time (Motink, 1993). The task is to identify the risk factors acting currently so that they can be managed effectively (Hanson & Bussière, 1996; Quinsey et al., 1995). There are a variety of sources of information and it is good practice to use as many of them as are available, as each has its own blend of strengths and weaknesses, and to remember that self-report by offenders can be particularly misleading. Less motivated offenders are likely to be anxious about the outcome of any interview and so may not be very truthful in their accounts of their offences. Even well-motivated offenders usually have a very different perception of their behaviour from that of their victims (Grubin & Wingate, 1996).

The preliminary assessment gathers information about the client's personal, sexual and offending history. This should include as much detail as possible about the previous and current offences, the name, age and gender of victims and the degree of violence used in carrying out the offences (Mander *et al.*, 1996).

The North West Regional Forensic Mental Health Service runs a community treatment programme for men who have sexually abused children. The risk assessment used has been adapted from that used in the sex offender treatment programme of the prison service. The following areas are reassessed at approximately two-monthly intervals:

- acceptance of guilt for the offence;
- minimization of consequences;
- insight into victim issues/empathy for victims;
- cognitive distortions;
- understanding of lifestyle dynamics;
- understanding of offence cycle;
- identification of relapse prevention concepts;
- disclosure of personal information;
- motivation to change behaviour.

Box 9.2

Acceptance of guilt for the offence

Very risky attitude or behaviour	Insists on his innocence; denies any participation in the offence.
Risky attitude or behaviour	Minimizes his role; attributes blame to victim, situation and others.
Minimum acceptable attitude or behaviour	Admits guilt and role as charged.
Appropriate attitude or behaviour	Fully admits guilt; exonerates victim of any blame or responsibility.
Most desirable attitude or behaviour	Admits guilt; recognizes deviant motivation for the offences.

THERAPEUTIC METHODS

An offender who is unable to accept that they have done anything wrong or unwilling to learn to take responsibility for their behaviour is unlikely to be motivated to make changes to reduce the likelihood of repeating the behaviour. It is difficult to engage someone in therapy if they maintain that they have not done anything wrong. On the other hand, someone who recognizes that they carried out their offences for their own sexual pleasure is in a stronger position to change.

CASE STUDY 9.1

When A began attending the group, he initially blamed his poor relationship with his wife for his sexual abuse of his stepdaughters. Two years later, he has recognized that he abused the girls because he was sexually attracted to them. He has since been able to work on using only appropriate sexual fantasies.

Box 9.3

Minimization of consequences

Very risky attitude or behaviour	Fully minimizes his role and any negative consequences.
Risky attitude or behaviour	Recognizes some effect but minimizes his role or the effect of his offending.
Minimum acceptable attitude or behaviour	Does not minimize the effects of his offending.
Appropriate attitude or behaviour	Does not minimize; thinks about the wide range of impact without minimization.
Most desirable attitude or behaviour	Does not minimize; actively accepts all the consequences of his offending.

Some offenders accept that they have committed offences against another person but do not accept the severity of the damage they have done to their victim. By acknowledging the full extent of the harm they have done and accepting all the consequences of their behaviour, offenders can demonstrate a growing maturity.

CASE STUDY 9.2

B believed that the boys he had abused had agreed to and enjoyed the sexual activity he had engaged them in. He could not accept that they had been harmed by his actions. Reading the statement of one of his victims severely shocked him and he has since been able to recognize how greatly affected the boy (now a young man) has been.

Box 9.4

Insight into victim issues/empathy for victim(s)

Very risky attitude or behaviour	No understanding of victim issues; sees little or no physical, mental stress or impact. Victims seen as unharmed or enjoying the abuse.
Risky attitude or behaviour	Some understanding but does not fully understand extent of physical/mental harm. Rationalizes that the victim is OK and no worse for the experience.
Minimum acceptable attitude or behaviour	Shows good understanding of victim issues relating to sexual abuse. Shows genuine empathy for the victim(s) of his offence(s).
Appropriate attitude or behaviour	Understands full extent of mental and physical harm and related impact on life. Shows full empathy with his victim(s).
Most desirable attitude or behaviour	Full understanding including long-term effects on victim's family, spouse, etc.

Being able to take the perspective of the victim is seen as an important development. Many men at the beginning of their treatment do not believe that they have harmed their victims. Many believe, to the contrary, that their victims have been helped by what other people choose to call abuse. Many offenders believe that their victims invited or enjoyed the sexual activity. They perceive ordinary childish friendliness as flirtation and ordinary childish curiosity as a desire for sexual activity with an adult. Many sex offenders fail to see their victims as people or fellow human beings; the children become simply the means of meeting the adult's own needs.

The use of audiotapes and videotapes is extremely effective in helping group members to develop insight into how victims/survivors of sexual abuse feel about their experiences. After the block of work on this topic, members are usually able to name a variety of problems encountered by victims. However, this tends to be an intellectual knowledge: the ability to recognize and empathize with the emotional impact usually comes later (if at all). Sometimes this block is due to the offender's own sexual victimization which they have not so far been able to accept. If this is so, it is necessary to offer some help with this in order to enable the group member to move on.

As group members progress they begin to develop a wider perspective on victim issues.

CASE STUDY 9.3

C had abused two of his stepdaughters, but there were six other children in the family. After his arrest, several of these other children wrote to him to say how much they missed him. The boys could not believe that their father had done anything bad and blamed their sisters for having their father taken away. In his early days in treatment, C was very angry with the social services department who refused to allow him to see his children. Over the following year, he began to reflect on the damage he had done to the relationships between the children and how he had provided such a dangerous role model of a violent and sexually abusive figure for his sons.

Box 9.5

Recognition of cognitive distortions

Very risky attitude or behaviour	Totally fails to understand the role cognitive distortions play in offending.
Risky attitude or behaviour	Partially recognizes cognitive distortions but sees them as only partially applicable.
Minimum acceptable attitude or behaviour	Recognizes role of cognitive distortions relating to sexual offending behaviour.
Appropriate attitude or behaviour	Recognizes personal use of cognitive distortions; avoids and/or challenges cognitive distortions.
Most desirable attitude or behaviour	Fully understands cognitive distortions; active change of current/past distortions regarding offences.

The ways in which offenders attempt to rationalize, excuse or justify their behaviour are called cognitive distortions. Offenders may believe that their victim initiated the sexual activity and many express the belief that their victim enjoyed what happened. This belief may even persist when, on closer questioning, they remember that the child struggled or cried. An offender can reduce his risk of reoffending by gaining insight into the methods he used to give himself permission to offend and remaining alert for signs of beginning to do so again.

CASE STUDY 9.4

D abused a little girl of 7. His view was that she was ugly and was lucky to have a man take a sexual interest in her.

E abused a nine-year-old. He believed that she was being abused by her brother and felt entitled to 'have some of that'.

F abused a number of boys and girls he enticed to his house by allowing them to play on his computer. Because the children returned to his house to use the computer, he was able to believe that they came back for more sexual activity.

G began his abuse of his granddaughters by tickling them. When they giggled he took it to mean that they were happy for him to touch them sexually. He was shocked when it was suggested that the girls giggled because they were ticklish or because they were embarrassed.

Box 9.6

Understanding of lifestyle dynamics

Very risky attitude or behaviour	Sees no relationship between his lifestyle and his sexual offending.
Risky attitude or behaviour	Has partial understanding of lifestyle and offence, but sees little or no need to change.
Minimum acceptable attitude or behaviour	Understands how his lifestyle relates to his offending.
Appropriate attitude or behaviour	Recognizes lifestyle dynamics; realizes need to change in future.
Most desirable attitude or behaviour	Recognizes lifestyle dynamics; actively seeks realistic ways to change.

At the beginning of their treatment, many offenders believe that their sexual offending is a problem only with their sexuality, which they would like to parcel off into a separate compartment and forget about. In fact, many aspects of their lives are involved in their offending behaviour. Many are able to identify stresses with which they were struggling when they were offending, for example money worries, relationship problems with adult partners or even an inability to gain or keep an adult partner. Many will also talk about having low or absent self-esteem or being depressed. Excessive drinking is not an uncommon method of trying to escape these problems. Clients who develop new, healthier, more adaptive strategies for dealing with their problems are less likely to act them out with illegal sexual behaviour.

CASE STUDY 9.5

H was sexually aroused by pubescent boys. He believed that his brain had been 'wrongly wired' and that, if this could be corrected, he would be 'cured' of his problems. He came to realize that his difficulties were much broader. His relationships with other people were based primarily on having his own needs met. He found it difficult to compromise or put the other person's needs first. He recognized that this bullying behaviour (though not sexual) was also abusive and began to try to change the way in which he related to other people.

J blamed his sexual abuse of his stepdaughters on his relationship with their mother. He has since been in a relationship with another woman. Many of the stresses present in his marriage are also present in this relationship but he is unable to see the similarities and therefore he is still subject to the same problems as before. Progress would mean that he began to recognize the pattern and try to order the relationship differently.

Box 9.7

Understanding of own offence cycle

Very risky attitude or behaviour	Denies the offence was anything more than a spontaneous act; no precursors/cycle.
Risky attitude or behaviour	Unable to identify cycle; may claim lack of memory or only partially applicable.
Minimum acceptable attitude or behaviour	Recognizes offence/deviant cycle and the relationship to his offending.
Appropriate attitude or behaviour	Identifies cycle as related to his offence; begins thinking how to change cycle.
Most desirable attitude or behaviour	Identifies cycle; actively seeks ways to avoid future offences.

Much work is done in helping offenders to discover their pattern (or cycle) of offending so that they can identify ways to break into it so as not to repeat it. This involves becoming aware of:

- the triggers (stresses or pressures) that led up to the offences;
- the role that sexual fantasies and masturbation played in planning or rehearsing the offences;
- how victims were selected, targeted and groomed;
- the cognitive distortions used to 'give permission' to offend;
- how the offender blocked out any feelings of guilt after committing the offences.

Box 9.8

Identification of relapse prevention concepts

Very risky attitude or behaviour	No understanding of relapse prevention concepts; unwilling to accept avoidance of high-risk thoughts or fantasies and high-risk situations.
Risky attitude or behaviour	Shows only partial or superficial understanding; cannot easily identify high-risk thoughts or fantasies and high-risk situations.
Minimum acceptable attitude or behaviour	Shows a clear understanding of relapse prevention concepts as applied to sexual offending.
Appropriate attitude or behaviour	Shows good understanding; actively able to relate concepts to his offence.
Most desirable attitude or behaviour	Fully understands proactive avoidance of high-risk thoughts or fantasies and high-risk situations.

The triggers that offenders identify include worries about money and jobs. They cite relationship problems and low self-esteem. By gaining insight into these elements of his behaviour and by learning new skills in these areas, an offender can begin to make appropriate changes in his life.

Relapse prevention techniques can play a key role in assisting offenders to reduce the likelihood of reoffending. These involve identifying their thought and behaviour patterns when they were offending so that they can be avoided.

High-risk thoughts can include feelings of being unwanted or unvalued or of supposed hurts by other people. Expected changes would be that the offender now tackles the problems directly instead of acting out sexually.

High-risk fantasies would be those involving, primarily, illegal sexual activities. Nurses working with sex offenders in a structured programme encourage group members to use fantasies that are about consenting sex with an age-appropriate adult partner, that each partner should be equally active and that the sex should be in the context of a loving relationship rather than a one-night stand. Nurses can discourage fantasizing about bondage or sadomasochism with a passive partner. Masturbating when angry or about someone the group member is angry with are also to be avoided. Similarly, the use of pornography should be discouraged. These things are clearly not necessarily illegal but are felt to be a special risk to men who have already shown a propensity to offend sexually as they allow sexual partners to be seen as objects rather than real people like the men themselves.

High-risk situations are those which place the offender in a position in which he could reoffend. This will vary according to each individual's pattern of offending. Examples are avoiding parks and playgrounds, not babysitting, not entering into relationships with people who have children. Nevertheless, the fact that an offender can recognize high-risk situations does not mean that he will avoid them.

CASE STUDY 9.6

K is sexually attracted to girls between three and seven years old. He had found his victims by going to parks and playgrounds and knows that he should avoid these places. Nonetheless, he went out on several occasions and made straight for local parks. Now, he is not allowed out unaccompanied from the medium-secure unit where he is an inpatient.

L spoke about the dangers for him of using the local swimming pool. A few days later, he was seen at the local baths with his small son. When challenged, he blamed the two-year-old for wanting to go swimming and said that his son's presence would prevent him from abusing any other children. His partner claimed that it was her fault for asking him to take their son. Here we have not only an offender ignoring what he knows to be real dangers but the situation is compounded by his partner colluding with him.

Box 9.9

Disclosure of personal information

Very risky attitude or behaviour	Refuses to disclose personal information even if trivial and even when pressured.
Risky attitude or behaviour	Reluctantly discloses personal information which may be trivial or superficial.
Minimum acceptable attitude or behaviour	Willing to disclose personal information as necessary.
Appropriate attitude or behaviour	Willing to share most personal information and details.
Most desirable attitude or behaviour	Openly shares and discusses intimate information in an open and receptive manner.

Although sex offenders tend to be unreliable at reporting their own behaviour, the building up of trust throughout the therapeutic period is important. A client who refuses to share his thoughts and attitudes with staff makes it extremely difficult to carry out any risk assessment. On the other hand, if a greater degree of trust and openness can be established during treatment, the level of risk can be assessed with greater ease.

CASE STUDY 9.7

M had established himself in a relationship with a woman who had a nine-year-old son. Consequently, the social services department had been involved in ensuring the safety of the child. M and his partner decided to have a baby. Neither of them discussed this with any of the professionals working with them until the pregnancy was well advanced, despite the important implications of their decision. Their action was a severe challenge to the trust that they wanted other people to put in them and raised serious quetsions about the woman's ability to protect her children.

Box 9.10

Motivation to change behaviour

Very risky attitude or behaviour	Not motivated to change; no perceived genuine interest in changing behaviour.
Risky attitude or behaviour	Motivation to change but inconsistent, transient or inappropriate reasons to change.
Minimum acceptable attitude or behaviour	Motivated to change behaviour.
Appropriate attitude or behaviour	Well motivated to change in a consistent and enduring manner.
Most desirable attitude or behaviour	Consistently well motivated to change for the safety of others; actively encourages other group members.

The changes that a sex offender has to make to his life can be far-reaching and painful. They are unlikely to be carried through where the client does not recognize their importance for himself. Most sex offenders enter therapy initially because they have to. They frequently express much self-pity: they have lost family, home, job or liberty. They bitterly regret these consequences of their behaviour. While this reaction is an understandable and reasonable starting place, one cannot assume long-lasting motivation to make the difficult changes needed. As members progress through treatment and gain understanding and insight, they develop more stable and stronger motivation to change.

CASE STUDY 9.8

N came to the group originally as a condition of bail wanting to avoid a prison sentence. He made no secret of planning to leave as soon as he legally could. During treatment, he recogized the far-reaching changes he needed to make in his personal life and now expresses a desire (believed by the group therapists to be genuine) to avoid damaging any more children.

CONCLUSION

Risk assessment and management with sex offenders is a daunting task and not one that can be undertaken in isolation. Communication between all the agencies involved is fundamental to effective working, especially in relation to offences against children. This raises the question of confidentiality: can sex offenders expect the same level of confidentiality from health care workers as other service users? The Royal College of Nursing document *Protecting Children* (RCN, 1997) is clear: 'Although parents and children have a general right to expect the information they give to nurses to be treated with respect and confidence, this does not automatically apply in cases of child abuse' (p.5).

Within therapeutic programmes with sex offenders, clients need to be warned (and reminded from time to time) that information they give will be shared with the other agencies working with them or their families and with the police if necessary. Although it could be argued that this may limit the openness of clients, it is felt to be the appropriate way to bear witness to the seriousness of the offences. In any situation where there may appear to be a conflict between the interests of a child and those of an adult, the child's welfare must always be given priority.

Many people have great concerns about sex offenders. Some feel that they should be locked away forever, never to see the light of day again. Within our liberal democracy this is not a feasible option. Therefore, it is important that at least some professionals develop skills in assessing and treating sex offenders so that the risks they pose to other members of society can be adequately and safely managed.

REFERENCES

Faulk, M. (1988) Dangerousness. In: M. Faulk (ed) *Basic Forensic Psychiatry*. Oxford: Blackwell, pp. 264–276.

Finkelhor, D. (1986) *A Sourcebook on Child Sexual Abuse*. Newbury Park: Sage.

Fisher, D. (1994) Adult sex offenders. In: T. Morrison, M. Erooga & R. Beckett (eds) *Sexual Offending Against Children*. London: Routledge, pp. 1–25.

Grubin, D. & Wingate, S. (1996) Sexual offence recidivism: prediction versus understanding. *Criminal Behaviour and Mental Health*. 6:4, 349–359.

Hanson, R.K. & Bussière, M. (1996) Sex offender risk factors – a summary of research results. *Forum on Corrections Research*. 8:2, 10–12. (Internet source: [http://198.103.98/crd/forum/e082/e082c.htm] 15th October 1997)

Lotke, E. (1996) *Issues and Answers – Sex Offenders: Does Treatment Work?* (Internet source: [www.ncianet.org.ncia/sexo.html] 12th January 1998)

Mander, A., Atrops, M., Barnes, A. & Munafo, R (1996) *Initial Recidivism Study – Executive Summary*. Anchorage: Alaska Department of Corrections. (Internet source: [www.uaa.alaska.edu/just/reports/9602sotp.html] 12th January 1998)

Marshall, P. (1997) *The Prevalence of Convictions for Sexual Offences*. Home Office Research Finding No. 55. London: Home Office Research and Statistics Directorate.

Motiuk, L.L. (1993) Where are we in our ability to assess risk? *Forum on Corrections Research*. 5:2, 45-60. (Internet source: [www.csc-scc.gc.ca/crd/forum/e052/e052f.htm] 8th December 1997)

Motiuk, L.L. & Brown, S.L. (1996) Factors related to recidivism among released federal sex offenders. Paper presented at the XXVI International Congress of Psychology, Montreal, Canada. (Internet source: [www.csc-scc.gc.ca/crd/reports/r48e/r48e/htm] 8th December 1997)

Quinsey, V., Rice, M. & Harris, G. (1995) Actuarial prediction of sexual recidivism. *Journal of Interpersonal Violence*. 10, 85–105.

Royal College of Nursing (1997) *Protecting Children*. London: RCN.

Vancouver Society for Male Survivors of Sexual Abuse (1995) (Internet source: [www.vcn.bc.ca/vsmssa/about.html] 16th October 1997)

Webster, C. (1995) The prediction of dangerousness and the assessment of risk in mentally and personality disordered individuals. Paper presented at Leciester University study seminar, organized by the Faculty of Law, Southampton University.

PART THREE

SPECIAL CONSIDERATIONS FOR MENTAL HEALTH NURSES WHO MANAGE CRISIS AND RISK

10 RISK ASSESSMENT IN THE CONTEXT OF MENTAL HEALTH CARE: SOME MORAL CONSIDERATIONS

Steven D. Edwards

RISK AND RISK ASSESSMENT

As I understand it, put as simply as possible, risk assessment in the context of mental health care is part of a programme of therapeutic management or care. The purpose of such management is to prevent clients from going into crisis, which can be defined as 'the point at which an undesired outcome becomes highly likely or has occurred' (Ryan, 1997, personal communication). The term 'management' applies to both the initial stages of risk assessment and the phase during which the service user is monitored or, less contentiously, remains in a therapeutic relationship with relevant health care professionals.

Hence, suppose a person with a history of mental health problems is about to leave hospital following an acute period of illness. Suppose further it is thought that the person may behave in ways which are harmful either to themselves or to others at some point after they leave hospital. In such circumstances, a risk assessment may be undertaken prior to the person leaving hospital and a programme of risk management devised. As noted, the purpose of all this is to prevent deterioration in the person's mental health and to prevent harm befalling the person, themselves or others.[1]

Risk assessment is used with clients for whom it is judged probable that they are vulnerable to harm themselves or others and that the degree of probability is above that to which all humans are constantly exposed. So the level of risk for which a risk assessment is considered appropriate must be above that to which all humans are exposed, otherwise people with mental health problems might properly claim they are being unfairly singled out for 'special' attention or scrutiny of their lifestyle.[2]

It can be claimed that the risks we all face merely by virtue of being alive typically fall into two types which seem separate. There are risks which are voluntarily undertaken, such as those which accompany activities such as mountain climbing, boxing and heavy smoking and drinking and more mundane but still voluntarily chosen risks involved in any life of even moderate activity, such as crossing a road, eating meat or living near an airfield. And also, there are unavoidable risks to which one is always susceptible, for example plane crashes, earthquakes and 'acts of God'.

It should be said, however, that there are real difficulties in separating these two categories of risk. The first category seems voluntarily chosen and the second unavoidable but clearly, a person's voluntarily chosen risks can increase the risk of susceptibility to the unavoidable risks. If one chooses to fly a great deal, it seems more likely that one will be involved in a crash than if one chooses never to fly. If one chooses to work extremely hard and subject oneself to high stress levels, one's risk of developing a health problem increases. So it can be problematic to separate voluntarily chosen from unavoidable risks.

Another way to reach this same conclusion is to argue that voluntarily chosen risks themselves stem from circumstances over which the person has little control and, hence, that the degree of voluntariness in such 'choices' is much less than widely thought. So choosing to smoke seems a voluntary choice, yet most smokers are females and from economically poorer sections of society. This can be taken to suggest that such choices are voluntary in a qualified sense only.

A further problem with the appeal to risk in a therapeutic context is that it seems inevitably to involve a supposition that the degree of risk to which an individual is subject can be specified. This is a major and controversial presupposition. Mental health problems surely differ for each individual. The *experience* of illness may differ between individuals, as may their individual responsivity and reactions to therapeutic interventions, their social circumstances and, indeed, the skills and interests of the health care professionals with whom they come into contact. These variables call into question the very possibility of specifying the degree of risk to which an individual is susceptible. Given this, it is not surprising that health care professionals' predictions of risk, for example of violent behaviour in clients, are often inaccurate (Ryan, 1994, 1996).

Another point concerning the concept of risk in the health care context runs as follows. Very crudely, it is common to point to a distinction between descriptive (fact-stating) and evaluative (value-stating) discourse (Hume, 1739/1978). The suggestion is that whilst there are means of resolving disputes concerning matters of fact (e.g. empirical evidence), no such means exist in the resolution of disputes in matters of value. Hence, to show that a concept is essentially evaluative calls into question the possibility of secure judgement regarding the application of that concept. For example, to show that the concept 'good' is essentially evaluative signals the possibility of irresolvable conflict in judgements concerning what is good. Hence, whilst Smith might think strawberry ice cream is good, Jones favours chocolate ice cream and there is no means to judge who is 'correct', that is, to determine which is 'really' the most good: strawberry or chocolate ice cream. The judgements of Smith and Jones simply reflect their evaluative preferences. Similarly, in aesthetic judgements, whilst Smith might favour Mozart, Jones favours Stockhausen and there is no means of resolving the question of who 'really' is the best composer. This can also be in moral discourse to show that, just as in matters of taste and aesthetics, there is no moral perspective from which to evaluate rival moral claims.[3] This generates a kind of scepticism concerning the possibility of making secure judgements in evaluative matters.[4]

The point of drawing attention to the distinction between descriptive and evaluative discourse is this. It seems plain that the concept of risk, as it features in the health care context, is inherently evaluative. For what are being considered and weighed in risk assessment are situations defined by reference to, first, their desirability and, second, the degree of harm or benefit which will ensue from their occurrence. So in risk assessment, which looks at the likelihood of 'positive' or negative' events (e.g. health-promoting events or harm-producing events), the terms 'positive' and 'negative' simply reflect whether those events are desired or undesired. So the concepts of positive or negative risk are inherently evaluative as they reflect whatever outcomes or situations the practitioner, service user or some other party values.

Exactly parallel points can be advanced in relation to the concept of crisis since this too seems inherently evaluative. As Ryan's definition, quoted earlier, makes evident, crises are defined by reference to their undesirability whether this be from the perspective of the service user, practitioner or some other party . Hence, crisis is inherently evaluative.

If the above is accepted, a common distinction, considered to be of some importance, can be queried. The distinction is one between 'objective' and 'subjective' perceptions of risk, discussed in the following passage.

Following widespread publicity of a murder or other violent act by a person with a mental illness, the public perception of the likelihood of the risk occurring will increase, even though the likelihood is no greater in reality than it was before the event.

(Ryan, 1996, p.94)

Here it is suggested that a distinction can be made between perceived risk and actual risk yet such a distinction can be queried on three grounds. First, as we have seen, *all* risk is perceived risk, as risk assessment simply reflects desired and undesired outcomes. Hence, the very idea of risk has human perception built into it. Second, at least in the mental health context (and probably elsewhere), the quantity and variety of variables which can conceivably prompt action (or inaction) seem so vast as to render the possibility of quantifying degree of risk for an individual service user extremely remote. Third, a difference between two parties in their assessment of the degree of risk present in any particular situation might simply be viewed as a sign of a difference in value orientation, that is, given that risk specification is inherently value laden. That a particular possible event is viewed as a risk (as desirable or undesirable) simply reflects the values of the judger.

Before moving on to consider the ramifications of these points, it may be useful to summarize the two main claims advanced above. The first is that the very idea of risk specification for individual mental health clients seems highly dubious given the complexity and variation in relevant variables. And second, the concept of risk, along with that of crisis, is essentially evaluative.

SERVICE USER AUTONOMY AND RISK MANAGEMENT

A rather cautious position is now beginning to emerge according to which, risk specification merely manifests the values of the specifier. Situations in which risk assessment is undertaken without the views of the service user being taken into account seem simply to involve a crude form of value imperialism; the imposing of one set of values upon a weaker party (i.e. politically weaker). It also seems likely to generate a cautious, conservative approach to risk management in which the client's freedom to make life choices is restricted on the grounds that they *might* harm either themselves or someone else. In this kind of situation, health care professionals act paternalistically, motivated by intentions to promote the well-being of the client but in which the client's own views are held to be largely irrelevant.

Paternalistic actions are not inherently unjustifiable. Parents act paternalistically toward their offspring and, mostly, their actions are perfectly justifiable when considered from the moral perspective. If a person (say, a very young child) is not able to choose how to live well or even safely, it seems perfectly legitimate to make a choice for that person in accordance with one's own standards of what makes a good or a safe life. When people are unable to take decisions concerning the conduct of their own lives, perhaps due to serious mental health problems, again it seems legitimate to make decisions for them according to one's own standards of what makes a good life.

However, when a person *is* able to make a decision concerning how they would like to live, in general such decisions are usually respected. This is a moral position which seems to have wide acceptance in Western cultures according to which, roughly speaking, people are entitled to choose their own ways to live, provided they do not impinge upon others' choices about how *they* wish to live. Regardless of whether one considers the life choices of another person wise or healthy, there is an obligation to respect such choices and not to impede their enactment. Such a position has been described as one in which the 'right' is more important than the 'good' (e.g. Sandel, 1984); that is, the right to choose how one wishes to lead one's life is considered more fundamental than whether one chooses a good life. In fact, the very notion of there being a good life for humans, that is, a way of living to which all humans should aspire, is rejected in this position in moral theorizing. What matters, above all, is that one has the 'right' to choose one's own conception of a good life and that one is not impeded from pursuing it.

This position, respected in our general dealings with each other, is also reflected in English law. For, as Mason & McCall Smith (1994) point out, under English law competent persons cannot legitimately be treated against their wishes, even in situations in which they will die unless treated. Moreover, if I understand her properly, such a position is positively endorsed by the nursing theory of Parse (1981).

So application of this moral theorizing to the mental health context implies that the therapeutic management of people with mental health problems should be restricted to periodically ensuring that the person remains capable of making their own life choices. Presumably, it would be envisaged that the intervals at which this checking takes place would be mutually agreed between the service user and the relevant health care professional, perhaps as may be stated on a so-called 'crisis card'. Hence, such a role includes only the assessment of the risk of the client's becoming ill again and losing their capacity for autonomous decision making. Even f it is judged that the level of risk is increasing, intervention would not be possible unless either sanctioned by the service user themselves (again, perhaps on a 'crisis card') or at the point at which the client's mental health deteriorates to the extent that their capacity for competent judgement is seriously compromised.

This is clearly a limited role but, as we have seen, it accords with a moral position reflected in the law and has independent plausibility (Edwards, 1996). It still involves behaving towards those with a history of mental health problems in ways which differ from those without such a history. Hence, it may be thought objectionable on the grounds that it unfairly discriminates against people with a history of mental health problems. Evidently, the decision-making capacities of most people are not monitored by a mental health care professional.

But even this quibble can be overcome if, as mooted earlier, the service user agrees on the details of the monitoring/management process. This has some similarities to the Care Programme Approach to risk management but it differs from such an approach mainly in that the service user would choose which, if any, relatives should be involved in the plan of care.

Although this approach to risk management is informed by a widely held position within moral theory, it has at least three well-known difficulties. First, the inclusion of mental health professionals in the risk management or monitoring process hinges upon the supposition that the service user agrees to such involvement. Plainly, not all clients would agree. So there is a key difficulty in implementing this model. The service user may simply decide that they prefer to risk becoming ill again rather than suffer the violation of privacy incurred by the monitoring of their mental state whilst they are well.

Second, problems arise if the mental health care professional judges that the service user is becoming unduly self-neglectful. The service user may be drinking excessively, drug taking, not socializing, not eating and not maintaining even minimally decent standards of personal hygiene. The 'autonomy-based' model allows that people can choose the lifestyles they wish, provided they do not impinge upon the autonomy of others. So this self-neglect could not justifiably be stopped unless it clearly stemmed from the client's loss of autonomy or it impinged upon the health of their neighbours, such as by causing pest infestation.

Third, and related to the last problem, it seems to follow from the autonomy-based model that even intentions to commit suicide would have to be respected. Can that be a plausible position? I do not propose to answer this question, save to add that it is undoubtedly a serious difficulty for the autonomy-based line that it has this final implication. It should be said, though, that the problems the position faces in relation to suicidal intentions need not render it wholly implausible. It might still be properly and justifiably applied to other aspects of health care work.

ANOTHER VIEW: MODERATED AUTONOMY

Among the merits of the autonomy-based approach is that it can help to guard against, or at least highlight, undue or excessive paternalism on the part of health care professionals. The approach stresses that risk management might simply impose a set of values on people who may be weak and vulnerable. To some extent, this can be avoided by using the Care Programme Approach in which it is ensured that 'all parties, including the person with the mental illness, are drawn together to agree a plan of care' (Ryan, 1996, p.101). However, even this seems unduly paternalistic in that, presumably, 'all parties' may involve people whom the service user would prefer to be absent. In any event, some of the problems with this approach seem serious, including problems arising from extreme self-neglect and the expression of suicidal intentions.

These *are* serious problems and it is highly implausible for health care professionals simply to 'respect the autonomy' of clients who are extremely self-neglectful or suicidal. One suggestion may be to question the weight of the attachment to the value of autonomy which the autonomy-based position seems to require. Although autonomy is of great importance, other values are also important, including those of care and benevolence. These seem of particular relevance to health care professionals since it is these which motivate their practice (officially, at least). Hence, references to a 'duty of care' have a particular significance. 'Care' in this context is supposed to involve a deep moral commitment, not simply a shallow kind of 'caretaking' (see, for example, de Raeve, 1996). This explains in part the difficulties involved in accepting a position in which autonomy is given such great weight. It seems to require that mental health care professionals simply suspend their caring commitment to clients. This seems, again, strongly counterintuitive and to place too little recognition on values other than autonomy.

A more abstract and important criticism of autonomy-based positions runs as follows. It is claimed that the autonomy-based line derives from a view of the self which is untenable. The autonomy-based position is said to conceive of selves as 'atoms', the natures of which are wholly independent of the social context in which they are located. Given this view of what it is to be a 'self', an autonomy-based position seems to follow: selves should simply have the right to choose their own conception of the good life. In criticism of this, it is argued that selves are, at least in part, socially constituted and, moreover, that this has certain ramifications for the moral dimension of our lives. The claim that selves are socially constituted seems highly plausible. Suppose, for example, one is asked who one is. Typically (necessarily?) one begins with one's name, but clearly this is not an adequate answer to the question. Further information such as one's place of birth or residence and some information regarding one's occupation or interests goes some of the way towards saying who one is (MacIntyre, 1981). According to what has become known as a narrative view of the self, selves are constituted by a narrative and this narrative, of necessity, involves reference to social factors (Edwards, 1997).

Further, as noted earlier, this view of what it is to be a self appears to bring with it certain implications for the moral dimension of human experience. The reason is that, according to the narrative account, selves are defined by reference to social elements, including relations with others such as family, friends and employers. But each of these kinds of relations has an inescapable moral dimension o it. One's relations to one's family can be described in purely biological terms, but what is important about them is their moral aspect. Social relationships both entail and are defined by reference to moral obligations. This engenders a different view of morality from that which follows from the atomistic account of the self. Selves are embedded in networks of social relations and these relations have a moral dimension to them (for example, see Larrabee, 1993). Hence a position is sketched which motivates and explains the weight attached to the values of benevolence and care.

Of course, the position has weaknesses and is in need of further development but the problems with the autonomy-based line described above seem severe enough to warrant careful consideration of rival positions. That described above allows a prominent role for the kinds of moral considerations which seem crucial to a regime of risk management which is infused with care, where 'care' signifies a commitment to the well-being and welfare of service users.

NOTES

1 Of course, it should not be supposed that risk management takes place only in the community context.

2 It may be pointed out that there is an important role for 'positive' risk-taking also. Hence, risk management should not be seen exclusively in terms of preventing harms (Ryan, 1996, p.104). However, against this, it can be pointed out that even negative risk management can plausibly be regarded as therapeutic and therefore positive, since its aims are to make it less likely that the service user will be in need of future mental health care interventions.

3 And, of course, Szasz (1972) famously exploited the evaluative nature of the concept of mental illness to argue against its legitimacy.

4 For a sound argument against its applicability to the moral sphere, see Taylor (1989).

REFERENCES

de Raeve, A.L. (1996) Caring intensively. In: H. Upton & D. Greaves (eds) *Philosophical Problems in Health Care*. Aldershot: Avebury, pp. 9–22.

Edwards, S.D. (1996) *Nursing Ethics: A Principle-based Approach*. London: Macmillan.

Edwards, S.D. (1997) The moral status of intellectually disabled individuals. *Journal of Medicine and Philosophy*. 22, 29–42.

Hume, D. (1739/1978) *A Treatise of Human Nature*. Oxford: Oxford University Press.

Larrabee, M.J. (ed) (1993) *An Ethic of Care*. London: Routledge.

MacIntyre, A. (1981) *After Virtue*. London: Duckworth.

Mason, J.K. & McCall Smith, R.A. (1994) *Law and Medical Ethics*, 4th edn. London: Butterworth.

Parse, R.R. (1981) *Man-Living-Health*. New York: John Wiley.

Ryan, T. (1994) The risk business. *Nursing Management*. 1: 6, 9–11.

Ryan, T. (1996) Risk management and people with mental health problems. In: H. Kemshall & J. Pritchard (eds) *Good Practice in Risk Assessment and Risk Management*, Volume 1. London: Jessica Kingsley Publications, pp. 93–108.

Sandel, M. (1984) The procedural republic and the unencumbered self. *Political Theory*. 12, 81–96.

Szasz, T.S. (1972) *The Myth of Mental Illness*. London: Paladin.

Taylor, C. (1989) *Sources of the Self*. Cambridge: Cambridge University Press.

11 MENTAL HEALTH SERVICE USERS AND RISK

Martin Hird and Keith Cash

INTRODUCTION

The imperative to involve service users in assessment has been stated in many mental health policies, charters and directives over the last decade. The importance of assessment processes that include the 'active participation' of both users and carers was stressed in *Caring for People* (Secretaries of State for Health and Social Security, 1989). More recently, the *Patient's Charter* (Department of Health [DoH], 1997a) has emphasized the importance of user involvement in choices about the services they use and the treatment they receive. The influential *Building Bridges* (DoH, 1996) states that: 'All aspects of the care planning process should involve the user' (3.1.2.). The new administration has reaffirmed these principles in the recent White Paper on primary health care (DoH, 1997b). For nurses, the *Code of Conduct* has raised an expectation that nurses will routinely involve service users in risk assessment. The principle is that a nurse must work in an open and co-operative manner with service users and carers, encourage their independence and involve them in the planning and delivery of care (United Kingdom Central Council, 1992, 1996).

In all the above documents users and carers are frequently linked. Historically, these groups have in common their lack of real power and involvement in clinical processes that is now rightly being challenged. However, they need to be separated both for conceptual reasons and for the practical purposes of consultation and involvement. In the case of risk assessment, for example, in rare situations the carer may be at risk from the service user or in other situations the carer may fear for the service user's safety when the latter has no such concerns.

Furthermore, a key concept in risk assessment is whether or not the service user's judgement about their risk taking or dangerousness is to be taken as valid. This is predicated on the idea that some groups of people do not have the capacity to make such judgements for themselves. This idea is commonly applied to specific groups of people, for example children, people with a learning disability and people with a mental illness. However, carers, as a group, are commonly seen to have this capacity, as are service providers. Because of this the latter groups are more likely to form alliances, at the level of a shared conception of a problem if not at the level of a shared plan of action. For these reasons this chapter will focus on service user involvement in risk assessment, rather than both user and carer involvement.

This concept of capacity to provide informed consent is expanded in the *Mental Health Act (1983) Code of Practice* (DoH and Welsh Office, 1993; see Chapter 15). This provides guidelines for determining the capacity for someone to

CASE STUDY 11.1

A mental health nurse working in the community is asked to assess Carol, a 61-year-old woman who is showing signs of self-neglect. She has said some 'odd things' to her GP that led him to make the referral. Her medical records inform the nurse that on a number of occasions Carol has assaulted staff in a hostel and on acute psychiatric wards where she has spent long periods of her adult life.

Over several visits the nurse experiences no threat from Carol, but observes that she lives in squalor and has signs of long-term self-neglect which are putting her health at risk. She regularly shouts at passers-by from her door and when walking back from the post office, often carries her money openly in her hand. The nurse is therefore concerned that Carol is at risk of victimization.

Carol herself reports no concern about the above risks and indeed states that, since leaving hospital, she has lived happily in her flat for several years with no problems. However, her main concern is that she believes a man in the flat above her can hear her conversations and has some malicious intent towards her.

Some issues for the mental health nurse
- What does *user involvement* in the risk assessment actually mean in the above scenario?
- At what levels in the system of health care delivery, of which the nurse is a part, can *user involvement* affect the course and outcome of this process of risk assessment and management?

weigh options in the balance and to make an informed choice at a particular point in time. The service user's right to autonomy and self-determination is therefore not absolute, having defined limits established by Parliamentary Act. If for this reason alone, the concept and practice of *involvement* in risk assessment is complex. However, the complexities increase when the ideas underlying user involvement are unpacked (see case study 11.1).

The remainder of this chapter explores the concepts that underlie user involvement, applies these to risk management and suggests some strategies for involvement. We will argue that the notion of user involvement is based on several different and not necessarily compatible perspectives and furthermore, that an understanding of these perspectives is essential if there is to be meaningful and genuine user involvement in the assessment of the risks that they face and/or pose.

PERSPECTIVES ON USER INVOLVEMENT

The literature about user involvement in mental health services refers to a range of theoretical perspectives that provide the rationale for involvement (Beresford, 1992; Thompson, 1995). Three main perspectives on user involvement can be identified: the protests of survivors, the rights of citizens and the choices of consumers. These strands can be traced historically. The first visible shoots of user involvement are recognizable in the 1960s when a number of forces coincided: the introduction of phenothiazine medication, the questioning of the medical model as a total explanation of personal distress (for example, Szasz, 1962), the birth of therapeutic communities (such as the Phoenix Unit in Oxford) and the multiplication of user-led campaign groups. Words which characterize this period are *conflict, oppression* and *democracy*.

In the 1970s and 1980s this protest matured into demands for equal rights of citizenship for sufferers of mental illness. This development took place at the same time as professional groups with expert knowledge were diversifying. It may be argued that the struggle for service users moved from a clash with those professionals following a medical model to a conflict with professional paternalism from all the range of experts (Rose & Rose, 1992). In this struggle, self-determination was seen as the goal for service users. Words like *paternalism, needs* and *rights* dominate in this period. In the 1990s the focus has moved to service users as consumers who have the same rights as consumers of other products in a market system. Key words which occur in this period are *quality, client satisfaction, consumer* and *choice*.

THE PROTESTS OF SURVIVORS

Though different and sometimes conflicting ideas belong to this section, they can be brought under the umbrella name of *antipsychiatry*. The unifying idea is a reaction against a medical model (or illness explanation) of people's distress. Key thinkers included Thomas Szasz (1962) who, from a libertarian stance, asserted that psychiatry was being used as a strategy for controlling social deviance and as such was an abuse of the power of medicine. Laing (1960), in contrast, criticized psychiatry from an existential position, redefining some mental illnesses as an adaptation of individuals to their circumstances. During the same period, the damning studies by Barton (1959) and Goffman (1961) of the total institutions in which psychiatry was predominantly practised were becoming known.

This combination of assaults on psychiatry has fuelled a rumbling protest since then. The literature on user involvement and publications of the various groups of service users are peppered with themes drawn from antipsychiatry (Barker & Peck, 1987). Issues such as the applicability of the medical model to personal distress, requests for increased emphasis on non-medical aspects of problems and scepticism about physical treatment of 'mental illness' all rely on assumptions that mental distress is not explainable simply using a medical model.

The key theoretical issue that arises from this position for risk assessment is how the risks associated with mental health service users are constructed. For example, when service providers discuss risk, they are invariably referring to the risk of death from self-harm or the risk of harm to others inflicted by the service user. Moreover, they are considering these risks in the context of protecting against the risk to themselves of litigation. There are, however, other dimensions

of risk, which may have a different weighting for the service user (Ryan, 1998)
For example, these include the risk to self-esteem from loss of autonomy, the risk
from medical treatments and the risk to self from violence or sexual victimization
on a hospital ward.

In case study 11.1, the service providers considered the probability very high
that Carol would suffer serious harm from her neglect of hygiene or from assault
by members of the public. Carol recognizes these risks but, in her evaluation: '
would rather die happy at home than in some ward or hostel'. Her felt need, in
contrast, is for protection from this man upstairs, though she is unable to define
exactly the threat he poses. Being poorly defined, this risk is, even after some
weeks of visiting, hard for the nurse to understand. Whose definition of risk
should prevail? In a plan of risk management, Carol wishes to emphasize risk from
the man upstairs and risk of loss of quality of life should she go into hospital.

THE RIGHTS OF CITIZENS

Larry Gostin's writings in the mid-1970s mark the first, well-argued, popular
rights-based justification for user involvement in mental health services (Gostin
1975). This perspective on user involvement may also be described as a quest for
the acquisition of equal rights of citizenship for mental health service users. It may
be argued that a person has the right to full self-determination in all cases except
when power must be exercised over them to prevent harm to others (Mill, 1962)
Such a stand would mean that to overrule someone's right to self-determination
for what is believed to be their own good is not justifiable. This right is protected
in United States law by the Patient Self Determination Act (1990) which establishes
that patients have the right to receive treatment by informed consent and to accept
or reject medical treatment. Moreover, the World Health Organization has 10
basic principles against which to measure the quality of mental health services,
those relevant to this discussion being the right to self-determination and the right
to be assisted in self-determination.

In contrast to this, it has been argued that the National Health Service is
established on the foundation of *enlightened paternalism* (Klein & Lewis, 1974).
For example Lipsedge (1995) states in the conclusion of an article on clinical risk
management that:

> *Mental health professionals have to accept that the practice of psychiatry is
> essentially a paternalistic activity, and that imposing a treatment against
> someone's will is justified when they believe that the patient's life or health
> would be at risk if coercion were not applied and the situation were allowed to
> deteriorate.*

(p.127)

Such a position may be challenged by the argument that taking risks with life and
health is accepted to be a part of normal life for non-service users. For example,
two individuals, say a rock climber and a smoker, may each look at the other and
argue for control of the other's activities while defending their own freedoms. So

service providers may have notions of harm and benefit (and their balance) which conflict with those of the service user. An example would be a case of a depressed person stating their intention to kill themselves.

Most people would concede that the level of control exerted by professional carers may legitimately vary from one type of clinical encounter to the next. Myers & MacDonald (1996), in looking at the assessment process, highlight the key dilemma of the process as that of balancing rights against risks. The key theoretical issues in this case concern the rights of the service user undergoing risk assessment; what degree of self-determination in their treatment is legitimate? Beresford (1992) refers to this dimension of involvement as the service user's voice. If it is accepted that this voice needs to be heard as part of risk assessment, what rights does this voice have and what are the resultant obligations on service providers? What rights has Carol to take the risks with her health specified above? Has she any rights to a service to help her manage the risk she perceives from the man upstairs?

THE CHOICES OF CONSUMERS

A development of the above dimension is the perspective of the service user having rights as a consumer. This was related to two developments: the spread of a market philosophy into the UK public sector and the general change in structure of the economy from a pattern of mass production and mass consumption to one of segmented marketing and more flexible forms of production and product. A key idea emerging from this was that expressed by Peters & Waterman (1982): that the best companies are close to their customers. Applying these ideas to mental health care gives us an image of a service user behaving much as a shopper: making choices, withholding favour from poor products and demanding products in short supply. Their involvement is as an 'active and informed citizen, able to demand the kind of health service he or she demands' (Higgins, 1992, p.6). The suppliers (providers) in turn, are intently looking at the service user, seeking their views on services and responding to expressed need. So the influential review *Working in Partnership* (DoH, 1994) stated that 'The principle of user and carer choice needs to be firmly established as a basis for the practice of mental health nursing' (p.9).

A number of objections may be levelled at this perspective. For some people, looking from an antipsychiatry standpoint: 'Survivors of the mental health system are no more consumers of mental health services than cockroaches are consumers of Rentokil' (Barker & Peck. 1987, p.1). This is because service users often have not made the choice to become consumers of mental health services in the first place. Due to their emotional, physical and psychological problems, they may not have the capacity to act as fully rational and informed customers (Friedson, 1994). Services are predominantly centred on need as defined by professionals, rather than on the individually defined wants of consumers (Barnes & Wistow, 1992).

Fisher (1992) argues powerfully that the language of *voluntariness* is misused in health and social care for the reasons presented above and that choice is usually limited to whether or not to receive care. In the case of risk management, even this final choice may be removed. Risk management could indeed be described as a process of removal of choices rather than facilitating and responding to service users' choices. To follow the consumer metaphor, therefore, in the case of risk assessment, the service user is like a potential consumer entering a shop – once in the shopkeeper locks the door and goes into a back room to discuss with their fellow shopkeepers whether or not to let the consumer out again without making a purchase.

The key theoretical issue is the extent to which the service is centred on enabling and responding to the choices service users make and the preferences that they state. To what extent, then, is the nurse in our case study to note and respond to Carol's choices and expressed needs only? Is Carol the consumer of the nurse's service or is it the GP, the taxpayer or society at large?

RISK ASSESSMENT AS REALITY NEGOTIATION

So far we have concentrated on the historical development of user involvement and the theoretical concepts which are variously included in it and we have raised questions about its relationship with risk assessment. There are a number of campaigning groups that seek to represent service users that use the above perspectives to varying degrees. From the above, it can be seen that it can be difficult, if not impossible, to arrive at a consensual position on the way that users can be involved in risk assessment. This means that the different groups have adopted varying positions with respect to service providers and the models that they employ. These positions vary from a close alliance with the medical model and with a carer's perspective, in the case of the National Schizophrenia Fellowship, to hostility to mainstream psychiatry and close alliance with those who have had negative and damaging experiences of mental health services, in the case of Survivors Speak Out. Consensus between these groups is not to be assumed and this suggests that user involvement will complicate rather than simplify decision making about resource allocation and directions for service development (Beresford, 1992). However, whether taken as groups or individually, the assessment of need from the expressed view of the service user is 'one of the most neglected areas in mental health services research in the UK' (Carter et al., 1995, p.385).

Given the problems of seeking the user's view by consulting with representative groups we will argue that a focus at a micro level, the level of involvement of the individual service user in their own risk assessment, is the most fruitful approach. Promoting service user involvement at this level can lead to challenges to existing definitions of problems and solutions and hence the boundaries currently seen to define community care. Moreover, assessments in which service users participate will be very different processes from those which derive solely from the professional judgements and could provide the impetus for a process of bottom-up (re)thinking (Barnes & Wistow, 1992). This day-to-day involvement of service users in risk assessment is a relational process performed with a service user, rather han a technical procedure performed on a passive subject. This latter approach is ypified by a three-stage process of identification, analysis and control. The nterpersonal skills required of nurses can principally be defined as interviewing and observation. Such a model casts the service user in the role of a passive object of enquiry and control.

In contrast, the concept of risk can be seen as socially constructed (Berger & Luckman, 1967) and risk assessment is therefore a process of reality negotiation between two parties. Risk is not like temperature, for example, which can be measured objectively on a unidimensional scale. Instead, it is something on which different perspectives exist (Adams, 1995; Brewin, 1992). Given the various perspectives on user involvement described above, a strategy is needed that enables the reality of these to be recognized. This process of reality negotiation includes the meeting of two linguistic worlds (Fisher, 1992): that of the professional, 'expert' care provider, who is looking in on an individual in the midst of a subjectively known, potentially alarming and disabling immediate experience. The process of negotiation is weighted heavily in favour of the service provider (Friedson, 1994; Morral, 1996) who has the power to withhold treatment or, in some cases, to ensure that compulsory treatment be given. The provider has society's sanction to give 'expert' and therefore authoritative opinion, with the knowledge base and associated language serving to exclude the user from dialogue.

Seeing risk assessment as a relational process of negotiation means that a key variable in this process is the type of relationship that develops between the service provider and the service user. Indeed, the process of risk management will involve a number of decisions made in the context of a web of relationships, for example between the service user and their carer, primary health care team contact, members of a community mental health team and so on. Risk assessment and management are then interpersonal processes running through social interactions during the whole course of any mental health crisis. Arguably, in taking such a focus, we are also looking at the essence of mental health nursing which, it is commonly accepted, has an interpersonal process at its core (Barker *et al.*, 1994; Peplau, 1988).

RISK ASSESSMENT FROM WITHIN AN ALLIANCE

So far we have identified the nature of the process of risk assessment, along with two factors which affect its dynamic: the power imbalance and the different linguistic worlds of the two groups involved. Some of what has been said, though, is true for most mental health assessment processes. There are, however, key points to look at specifically affecting the dynamic of the relational process of risk assessment, which directly influence the service user's involvement. We have asserted that an important variable affecting assessment is the type of relationship between service provider and user. However, Eastman's (1996) summary of the *Confidential Inquiry into Homicides and Suicides by Mentally Ill People* (Steering Committee, 1996) identified key points compromising risk assessment. One of these was the lack of time for face-to-face contact with service users, an essential ingredient for a relational rather than observational process.

While time may be one factor, another is the process of practitioners distancing themselves from those who are perceived as potentially dangerous (Lakeman & Curzon, 1998). Such is the current awareness of and sensitivity to risk (real and imagined) that service providers are keeping a distance from service users, forming only impoverished relationships. Paradoxically, this may increase the risk of violence in service users (Whittington & Wykes, 1994) since service users, in turn, may hold back from more open discussion of issues surrounding risk because of fear of the consequences. Commonly accommodation or outpatient talking treatments may be withheld from those who are seen to be a risk to themselves or others. Service users who have deliberately harmed themselves refer to being punished or patronized and finding treatments barred to them when they present to services in crisis (Pembroke, 1996).

Moreover, other areas of need may be neglected in favour of those associated with the risk identified by the service providers. Echlin (1995), for example, notes that in the current climate risk reduction seems to be a higher priority than making those improvements in someone's quality of life which could sustain them in the longer term. Lastly, fear of litigation by service providers will often lead them to err on the side of caution and control rather than enabling and empowering in managing risk (Carson, 1996).

The above factors are some of the potent forces affecting the dynamic of this alliance between users and providers. It is significant that all the above dynamics work against the development of a close alliance between service users and providers.

PRACTICAL STRATEGIES TOWARDS SERVICE USER INVOLVEMENT

Up to this point we have avoided discussion of techniques for the involvement of service users in risk assessment because an understanding of the conceptual issues at the core of user involvement and risk assessment is essential for any successful involvement. Without this understanding, there is a very real danger of superficial and tokenistic involvement strategies being developed. Given the complexity of the processes of assessment and user involvement, it is not possible to produce a definitive or exhaustive manual of how to do it. Rather, some general guidelines can be given that will hopefully serve as a springboard for individual reflection on practice.

There are several stages in this process. The first is creating the context that providers of mental health services need to establish, as a foundation for the process of risk assessment, through widely publicizing the rights of the service users. A number of NHS trusts (for example, Bethlem and Maudsley NHS Trust, 1996) have provided a Charter of Rights based on and extending the *Mental Health Charter* (DoH, 1997a). These provide a knowledge of the ground rules for the service user entering an assessment that can both raise their expectations for involvement and provide a basis on which to challenge behaviour which falls short of the standards. These statements may need to include a declaration of the right to receive, and the obligation to provide, assessment and treatment to protect the safety of the service user along with the safety of the public when they may potentially be compromised by the behaviour of an individual believed to be suffering from a mental illness.

The second stage is the preparation that the nurse has undergone to make the assessment. Ellis (1993), in the conclusion of a study on service user and carer involvement in assessment, comments on the critical need for training to challenge practitioners to address issues of both value and power in their assessments. The substantial involvement of service users at all levels of nurse training would be an ideal means to reach that end and was recommended by the review of mental health nursing (DoH, 1994). To have real effect, the service users would ideally be involved in more than simply an occasional talk or discussion but rather in whole blocks of study, enabling an exploratory alliance between the student and the service user to be formed. The Pathfinder NHS Trust has taken positive well-publicized steps to promote the recruitment of service users as employees. Working alongside colleagues who have had experience of service use will challenge practitioners to address these issues of value and power in interventions (Davidson, 1997).

The third stage is addressing the issue of the balance of power between the provider and the user in the assessment interview, irrespective of whether the service user is seen alone or not. The place of advocates in assessment procedures is now accepted in principle but is patchy in actual practice. While paid and trained advocates may be in limited supply, anyone with whom the service user is comfortable can fill the role of fellow citizen and witness and this presence is likely to affect the type of alliance formed with the assessor.

The test of any strategy for user involvement is, of course, when there is an element of coercion or control applied by service providers. How can we practically talk about involvement in, for example, an assessment leading to the application for involuntary admission under the Mental Health Act (1983) or when a service user's statements about their intent not to harm someone are not believed? Fisher (1992), referring principally to social care, usefully draws a distinction between free and coercive agreements:

> *Where, however, social care is intentionally controlling, we must distinguish free from coercive agreements, and avoid converting the recipient of social care into the active consumer by 'word magic'. In many of these circumstances, the language of agreements is less accurate than that of sanction, denoting authority to take certain courses of action without implying freedom and power that the user does not possess.*
>
> (p.62)

The first practice to establish in circumstances in which self-determination is overruled is that any act of control needs to be done explicitly. When a level of explicit control has been taken service providers can involve service users by clear communication about the duration, nature and boundaries of their control. This communication ideally needs to be supported by a written record of the process outcome of the assessment and its implications for the service user. This recor serves to support the communication, but also gives the service user a basis t challenge aspects of the decisions at a later date. The taking of some control from service users does not mean the loss of all control and rights. As such, nurse providing care in inpatient areas need to be at the forefront of protecting th rights and dignity of detained people and maintaining involvement in therapeuti alliances even in an environment of control. The personal accounts of service user undergoing compulsory treatment are instructive, reserving fiercest criticism no for this act of control but for associated lack of care and respect from within tha relationship (see, for example, Pembroke, 1996). Needless to say, explici

---

Box 11.1

Strategies for user involvement in risk assessment

- Having assessments that explicitly identify and focus on the service user's expressed need and associated risk, but that have realistic mechanisms for integrating normative needs introduced by service providers into care planning.

- Ensuring that assessments are able to incorporate an understanding of the service user's perspective on risks they are facing, rather than on merely categorizing and quantifying risk. This means that the sort of risks being assessed have to be wider than those usually considered (harm to self or others) and include those of importance to service users such as deprivation, dependency and vulnerability (Ryan, 1998).

- Structuring assessments so that they look at strategies the service user already has for managing risk and using these as a starting point for planning risk management.

- Establishing plans that empower service users to recognize and respond to their own prodromal states and thus effectively pass on expertise and responsibility for risk management to service users. This means negotiating the lines of communication so that the user's knowledge of their own condition is not rejected or ignored by the other professionals they might approach.

- Developing self-management orientated risk management plans of care for some users, such as those described by the Manic Depression Fellowship (1995).

- The use of advanced directive care plans, in which service users and providers work together to produce plans of care for future mental health crises, in which compromised capability may limit full involvement in risk management such as the *Self Injury Treatment Checklist* (Pembroke & Smith, 1996).

---

communication during the process of restoration of self-determination needs to follow.

This principle is not limited to mental health practice. For example, in midwifery a birth plan for the delivery of a baby can be drawn up which includes a statement of the mother's preferences for the management of the various hazards of childbirth. However, complications may arise where the midwife or obstetrician needs to overrule the mother's preferences without negotiation or agreement, for example when the mother is unable to maintain her control and involvement in decisions due to exhaustion or intoxication from drugs. Good practice would suggest that the midwife or obstetrician later talk the mother through the birth and the decisions that were made, along with a rationale, and discuss the prospective birth plan for future children in the light of events. In taking this approach, the professionals can achieve a number of things: re-establish an adult–adult relationship, hand the birth experience back to the mother (which had been lost in the mist of intoxication and exhaustion), make the professional vulnerable to criticism, explicitly hand back responsibility for planning of possible future deliveries and allow learning to take place from the past experience.

How many community mental health nurses routinely seek an opportunity to debrief with service users on the ward following an assessment which has led to compulsory admission? How many of us as ward nurses hand experiences back to inpatients after they have been restrained or given medication against their wishes, thereby making ourselves vulnerable to criticism but re-establishing adult–adult relationships?

Lastly, we will consider service user involvement in by far the most common risk assessment and management situations: those in which the service user is able to safely maintain full self-determination. There is a common rhetoric of empowerment in much nursing literature but the practice of paternalism in assessment is more common (Savage, 1991) and in many cases the only real choice available to service users is whether or not to refuse the service (Cox, 1996). Good practice would involve the service user through a number of methods as outlined in Box 11.1.

CONCLUSION

We have considered risk assessment and management in relational terms; this is something we do with service users rather than to them. We have provided some practical examples as springboards to initiate other ideas on involvement. Lastly, to put this chapter in its place, our own nursing practice has been affected most strongly by reflecting on experiences of becoming vulnerable and needy oneself and by listening to and reading about the experiences of service users and *not* by reading chapters on user involvement.

REFERENCES

Adams, J. (1995) *Risk*. London: University College Press.

Barker, I. & Peck, E. (1987) *Power in Strange Places*. London: Good Practices in Mental Health.

Barker, P., Reynolds, W. & Ward, T. (1994) A critique of Watson's caring ideology: the proper focus of psychiatric nursing. *Journal of Psychosocial Nursing and Mental Health Services*. 32:5, 17–22.

Barnes, M. & Wistow, G. (eds) (1992) *Researching User Involvement*. Leeds: Nuffield Institute.

Barton, R. (1959) *Institutional Neurosis*. Bristol: J. Wright.

Beresford, P. (1992) Researching citizen involvement: a collaborative exercise? In M, Barnes & G. Wistow (eds) *Researching User Involvement*. Leeds: Nuffield Institute, pp.16–32.

Berger, P. & Luckman, T. (1967) *The Social Construction of Reality*. New York: Anchor Books.

Bethlem and Maudsley NHS Trust (1996) *User's Charter*. London: Bethlem and Maudsley NHS Trust.

Brewin, C.R. (1992) Measuring individual needs for care and services. In: G. Thornicroft, C.R. Brewin & J. Wing (eds) *Measuring Mental Health Needs*. London: Gaskell, pp. 220–236.

Carson, D. (1996) Risking legal repercussions. In: H. Kemshall & J. Pritchard (eds) *Good Practice in Risk Assessment and Management*, Volume 1. London: Jessica Kingsley Publications. pp. 3–12.

Carter, M.F., Crosby, C., Geertius, S. & Startup, M. (1995) A client-centred assessment of need. *Journal of Mental Health*. 4:4, 383–394.

Cox, J. (1996) An unwanted concept. *Nursing Standard*. 10:46, 24–25.

Davidson, B. (1997) Charting a new course. *Mental Health Nursing*. 17:4, 30–31.

Department of Health (1994) *Working in Partnership: A Collaborative Approach to Care*. London: HMSO.

Department of Health (1996) *Building Bridges: A Guide to Arrangements for Interagency Working for the Care and Protection of Severely Mentally Ill People*. London: The Stationery Office.

Department of Health (1997a) *Patient's Charter: Mental Health Services*. Leeds: Department of Health.

Department of Health (1997b) *The New NHS: Modern • Dependable*. London: The Stationery Office.

Department of Health and Welsh Office (1993) *Code of Practice: Mental Health Act*. London: HMSO.

Eastman, N. (1996) Inquiry into homicides by psychiatric patients: systematic audit should replace mandatory review. *British Medical Journal*. 313, 1069-1071.

Echlin, R. (1995) *Partners in Change*. London: King's Fund.

Ellis, K. (1993) *Squaring the Circle: User and Carer Participation in Needs Assessment*. York: Joseph Rowntree Foundation.

Fisher, M. (1992) Users' experiences of agreements in social care. In: M. Barnes & G. Wistow (eds) *Researching User Involvement*. Leeds: Nuffield Institute, pp. 47–64.

Friedson, E. (1994) *Professionalism Reborn: Theory, Prophecy and Policy*. Cambridge: Polity Press.

Goffman, E. (1961) *Asylums*. New York: Anchor Books, Doubleday.

Gostin, L. (1975) *The Rights Business*. London: MIND.

Higgins, R. (1992) Consumerism and participation. *Senior Nurse.* 12:5, 3–4.

Klein, R. & Lewis, J. (1974) *The Politics of Consumer Representation.* London: Centre for Policy Studies.

Laing, R.D. (1960) *The Divided Self.* London: Tavistock.

Lakeman, R. & Curzon, B. (1998) Society, disturbance and illness. In: P. Barker & P. Davidson (1998) *Psychiatric Nursing: Ethical Strife.* London: Arnold, pp. 26–38.

Lipsedge, M. (1995) Clinical risk management in psychiatry. *Quality in Health Care.* 4:2, 122–128.

Manic Depression Fellowship (1995) *Inside Out: A Guide to Self-Management of Manic Depression.* London: Manic Depression Fellowship.

Mill, J.S. (1962) *On Liberty and Utilitarianism.* New York: New American Library.

Morral, P. (1996) Clinical sociology and the empowerment of clients. *Mental Health Nursing.* 16:3, 24–27.

Myers, F. & MacDonald, C. (1996) Power to the people? Involving users and carers in need assessment and care planning – views from the practitioner. *Health and Social Care in the Community.* 4:2, 86–95.

Pembroke, L.R. (1996) *Self-Harm: Perspectives from Personal Experience.* London: Survivors Speak Out.

Pembroke, L.R. & Smith, A. (1996) *Self Injury Treatment Checklist.* London: National Self-harm Network.

Peplau, H. (1988) *Interpersonal Relations in Nursing.* London: Macmillan.

Peters, T. & Waterman, R. (1982) *In Search of Excellence.* New York: Harper & Row.

Rose, D. & Rose, N. (1992) The subject of psychiatry: power, participation and resistance. *Asylum.* 7:1, 17–18.

Ryan, T. (1998) Perceived risks associated with mental illness: beyond homicide and suicide. *Social Science and Medicine.* 46:2, 287–297.

Savage, P. (1991) Patient assessment in psychiatric nursing. *Journal of Advanced Nursing.* 16:3, 311–316.

Secretaries of State for Health and Social Security (1989) *Caring for People: Community Care in the Next Decade and Beyond.* London: HMSO.

Steering Committee of the Confidential Inquiry into Homicides and Suicides by Mentally Ill People (1996) *Report of the Confidential Inquiry into Homicides and Suicides by Mentally Ill People.* London: RCP.

Szasz, T.(1962) *The Myth of Mental Illness.* London: Secker & Warburg.

Thompson, J. (1995) *User Involvement in Mental Health Services: the Limits of Consumerism, the Risks of Marginalisation and the Need for a Critical Approach.* University of Hull: Research Memorandum No. 8.

United Kingdom Central Council (1992) *Code of Professional Conduct.* London: UKCC.

United Kingdom Central Council (1996) *Guidelines for Professional Practice.* London: UKCC.

Whittington, R. & Wykes, T. (1994) An observational study of nurse behaviour and violence in psychiatric hospital. *Journal of Psychiatric and Mental Health Nursing.* 1:1, 85–92.

12 THE ROLE OF PSYCHOPHARMACOLOGY IN MANAGING CRISIS AND RISK

Richard Gray

INTRODUCTION

Psychopharmacology plays a critical part in the prevention and management of risk. This chapter will examine treatment non-compliance and the use of medication in preventing and managing violent incidents and outline clinical practice guidelines for effective medication management.

Mental health crises often result directly from service users stopping their medication. Repeated studies have implicated treatment non-compliance as a crucial factor associated with relapse and rehospitalization (Green, 1988; Haywood *et al.*, 1995). Some studies have also demonstrated that treatment non-compliance is associated with violence in psychotic service users (Torrey, 1994). Indeed, in recent well-publicized tragic incidents involving people with schizophrenia such as Christopher Clunis, Anthony Smith, Raymond Sinclair and Martin Marcell, treatment non-compliance has been cited as a contributing factor. Rates of non-compliance of between 10% and 80% have been reported in various reviews of psychotic service users (Babiker, 1986; Young *et al.*, 1986). These variations can be attributed to different treatment settings (e.g. inpatient and outpatient) and methods of measuring compliance. Non-compliance rates of around 50% have been reported in service users with depression and other chronic physical disorders (Kemp & David, 1995).

Improved rates of compliance could dramatically reduce relapse rates and prevent many crisis situations occurring. Kissling (1994) suggests that good medication management may improve compliance and could potentially reduce the relapse rate to about 15% (currently around 50% of service users relapse within the first year of remission and about 85% do so within the first five years [Kemp *et al.*, 1997]). In order to improve compliance rates, it is first necessary to examine why service users are non-compliant.

FACTORS AFFECTING COMPLIANCE

In a comprehensive review of factors associated with non-compliance in psychotic service users, Kemp & David (1995) proposed that variables can be classified into those related to the illness, the treatment and the person.

Illness-related factors include lack of insight (Bartko *et al.*, 1988; Lin *et al.*, 1979; McEvoy *et al.*, 1989; van Putten *et al.*, 1976), symptoms (for example, paranoia, thought disorder, hostility, delusional beliefs about medication, grandiosity) (Appelbaum & Gutheil, 1980; Hoge *et al.*, 1990; Marder *et al.*,

1983; van Putten, 1974) and cognitive impairment (Geller, 1982; Macpherson *et al.*, 1996; Weiden *et al.*, 1986).

Factors associated with treatment include the side-effects of antipsychotics, for example akathisia, akinesia, neuroleptic dysphoria, sexual dysfunction, dystonias, tremor, rigidity and weight gain (Buchanan, 1992; Michaux, 1961; Nelson, 1975; van Putten, 1974; van Putten *et al.*, 1981; Weiden *et al.*, 1986).

Person-related factors include the individual's personality and sociocultural background. A number of studies have highlighted that antichemical and antipsychiatry views are common in society (e.g. Angermeyer & Matschinger, 1994). Beliefs about the benefits of 'alternative' cures (such as diet) and the role of self-control and willpower in overcoming the illness are also prevalent in society (Weiden *et al.*, 1986).

In order that effective clinical practice guidelines can be developed to help manage service user's medication more effectively and minimize crisis and risk, it is first necessary to examine how the drugs used to treat mental disorder work.

ANTIPSYCHOTICS AND NEUROLEPTICS

Chlorpromazine, the first effective drug for the treatment of schizophrenia, was introduced in 1953. Its success led to the introduction of many similar agents, known as conventional neuroleptics. Table 12.1 summarizes commonly used conventional neuroleptic drugs and their approved British National Formulary (BNF) dose ranges.

These drugs interact with a number of neurotransmitter systems within the brain. In schizophrenia, the most important of these are the dopaminergic and serotonergic pathways. Two of the principal dopaminergic pathways are the mesolimbic and nigrostriatal systems. Neuroleptics block dopamine D2 receptors in the mesolimbic pathway and it is thought that this is responsible for their efficacy against positive symptoms such as hallucinations and delusions (Richelson, 1984; Seeman, 1980; van Wielinck & Leysen, 1983). However, a similar level of dopamine receptor blockade in the nigrostriatal pathway produces extrapyramidal side-effects (EPS) such as akathesia, dystonia, parkinsonism and tardive dyskinesia (Haase, 1954, 1978). Gray *et al.* (1997) observe that conventional neuroleptics are

Table 12.1

Neuroleptic drugs and approved BNF dose ranges

Drug	Chemical group	BNF approved dose range (mg/day)
Chlorpromazine	Phenothiazine	25–1000
Thioridazine	Phenothiazine	150–600
Trifluoperazine	Phenothiazine	10–45
Haloperidol	Butyrophenone	1.5–200
Flupenthixol	Thioxanthene	6–18
Sulpiride	Benzamide	400–2400
Pimozide	Diphenylbutylpiperidine	2–20

also responsible for a variety of other side-effects, including sedation (mediated via blockade of histamine H1 receptors), anticholinergic effects (blurred vision, dry mouth, constipation, via blockade of muscarinic receptors) and raised prolactin levels (amenorrhoea, galactorrhoea, sexual dysfunction in males, via blockade of D2 receptors).

Despite revolutionizing the treatment of schizophrenia, conventional neuroleptics have a number of significant problems. These include a lack of efficacy in the treatment of negative symptoms and the failure of about 30% of service users to respond to treatment.

In 1988, Kane et al. demonstrated that a new drug, clozapine, could be used safely and effectively in treatment-resistant schizophrenia. Clozapine is the prototypical atypical antipsychotic and has repeatedly been shown to be effective in treating both the positive and negative symptoms of schizophrenia with a low incidence of EPS (Clozapine Study Group, 1993; Matted, 1989; Meltzer et al., 1989; Owen et al., 1989). Clozapine has a greater affinity for serotonin 5-HT2a receptors and the blockade of these is thought to be at least partially responsible for clozapine's improved efficacy.

Based on the serotonin-dopamine hypothesis, a new generation of novel antipsychotics has been developed. These include risperidone, sertindole, olanzapine, quetiapine and ziprasidone (Gray et al., 1997). These are as effective as haloperidol in the treatment of schizophrenia but have an improved side-effect profile.

PRESCRIBING AND ADMINISTRATION OF MEDICATION

A number of recent studies have looked at the prescribing and administration of psychiatric drugs, particularly antipsychotics (Chaplin & McGuigan, 1996; Cornwall et al., 1996; Hillam & Evans, 1996; Krasuck & MacFarlane, 1996; Newton et al., 1996; Yorston & Pinney, 1997). Poor prescribing of psychiatric medication may significantly increase the risk of unwanted side-effects and reduce rates of compliance.

In an audit of antipsychotic prescribing in Amersham Hospital in south Buckinghamshire, Yorston & Pinney (1997) reported that 7% of service users were prescribed doses of antipsychotic medication exceeding BNF recommended limits. Cornwall et al. (1996) audited the use of high-dose antipsychotic medication for service users admitted to an intensive care unit and reported that 9% were prescribed antipsychotic medication in excess of 1 g/day chlorpromazine equivalent. Krasuck & MacFarlane (1996) reported that in a review of 177 service users' drug charts at the Bethlem Royal Hospital in Kent, 7.3% were prescribed doses of antipsychotics in excess of 1 g/day of chlorpromazine equivalent.

Chaplin & McGuigan (1996) examined the case notes of 107 service users receiving antipsychotic medication at Springfield Hospital in London. The median dose of chlorpromazine equivalent prescribed was 756 mg/day. Doses in excess of BNF prescribed limits were recorded for 36.5% of service users. Hillam & Evans (1996) observed that 64.5% of service users in two London intensive care wards

Table 12.2

Antipsychotic medication prescribing data

Study	n	Setting	Average dose (chlorpromazine equivalent)	Percentage of patients exceeding BNF limits (including PRN)	Other information
Yorston & Pinney (1997)	226	Amersham Hospital, south Buckinghamshire	Not reported	7% (25%)	Polypharmacy common
Cornwall et al. (1996)	57	Locked intensive care unit, Newcastle upon Tyne	Not reported	9%	
Chaplin & McGuigan (1996)	107	Springfield Hospital, London	Median 756 mg/day	36.5%	Polypharmacy common
Krasuck & McFarlane (1996)	177	Bethlem Royal Hospital, Kent	Mean 297 mg/day	7.3% (21.9%)	
Hillam & Evans (1996)	93	2 London intensive care wards	Mean 2108 mg/day (including PRN)	64.5%	3% of patients prescribed 54 antipsychotics
Newton et al. (1996)	247	New Cross Hospital, Wolverhampton	Not reported	2%	

were prescribed doses in excess of BNF limits. These results are in stark contrast to findings by Krasuck & MacFarlane (1996) and Cornwall et al. (1996). Table 12.2 summarizes the data on the prescribing of antipsychotic medication.

The number of service users being administered high doses of antipsychotic varied dramatically between studies (2–64.5%). However, it is clear that a significant number (perhaps 20%) of service users are being administered doses of antipsychotics in excess of BNF limits. Such high doses may be given to help manage perceived or actual risk (such as violence), with the most disturbed and unwell service users being prescribed higher doses of medication. Whilst there is strong anecdotal evidence to suggest that this goes on in practice, the evidence to support the administration of high doses of antipsychotic medication to manage risk is inconclusive. The stark contrast between the percentage of service users on high doses of antipsychotics in London (64.5%; Hillam & Evans, 1996) and Newcastle (9%; Cornwall et al., 1996) seems to emphasize this point. Why should one intensive care unit use substantially higher doses of antipsychotics than another comparable unit?

MEDICATION MANAGEMENT

Increasing emphasis is being placed on the mental health nurse's role in helping service users to manage their medication. A number of recent studies have outlined the components of effective medication management (Bennett et al., 1995a,b; Gray & Smedley, 1996; Gray et al., 1997; Gray & Gournay, 1997). They include:

- an awareness of the adverse effects of medication and skills in detecting and managing these effects using reliable measures;
- skills in assessing psychopathology;
- the use of cognitive behavioural and educational interventions with both service users and their carers.

SIDE-EFFECTS

Assessment

In a series of studies, Bennett et al. (1991, 1995a,b) examined the nurse's role in monitoring the side-effects of antipsychotic medication. They sent a 20-item questionnaire to 55 community psychiatric nurses (CPNs) in three health authorities. CPNs generally reported that they were actively involved in the administration and monitoring of antipsychotic medication. Although 80% of CPNs felt that their education had adequately prepared them to monitor the side-effects of antipsychotic medication, results demonstrated that in practice they assessed only three or four of the 13 most common side-effects of antipsychotic medication. The side effects most commonly assessed were: parkinsonism, akathisia and dystonias. There was no evidence that CPNs used any standard measures to monitor side-effects. Despite the small sample size, this study does highlight that the side effects of antipsychotic medication are not being adequately monitored. A number of valid and reliable measures have been developed for the assessment of the side-effects of antipsychotics.

EPS may be assessed by a number of general rating scales or by scales which measure specific characteristics. General rating scales include:

- the Extrapyramidal Rating Scale (ESRS; Chouinard et al., 1980), widely accepted as a sensitive and reliable measure of EPS;

- the Targeting of Abnormal Kinetic Effects (TAKE) Scale (Wojckik et al., 1980);

- the Extrapyramidal Symptoms Scale (Adler et al., 1989);

- the UKU rating scale (Lingjaerde et al., 1987).

Parkinsonism can be measured using the Extrapyramidal Side Effects Rating Scale (EPSE; Mindham, 1976; Simpson & Angus, 1970). Diagnosis of akathisia involves questioning service users about their subjective experiences. This can be unreliable if used as the sole method of diagnosis, as akathisia may be mistaken for anxiety, agitation or psychotic excitement (van Putten & Marder, 1986, 1987). A reliable rating scale should help differentiate side-effects from behavioural disturbances. Two of the most popular scales for measuring akathisia are the Barnes Akathisia Rating Scale (Barnes, 1989) and the Hillside Akathisia Rating Scale (Fleischhaker et al., 1989).

Tardive dyskinesia (TD) is most commonly assessed using the Abnormal Involuntary Movement (AIMS) Rating Scale (Guy, 1976; Lane et al., 1985; Munetz & Benjamine, 1988). This provides a comprehensive assessment of involuntary movements at different body sites. Alternatively, TD may be assessed using the ESRS (Chouinard et al, 1980) or the Simpson/Rockland Scale (Simpson et al., 1979).

Use of these scales requires some degree of training. However, the Liverpool University Neuroleptic Side Effect Rating Scale (LUNSERS) can be completed by service users and administered by health care professionals without specialized training. The LUNSERS (Day et al., 1995) is a 51-item self-report scale covering the psychological, neurological, autonomic, hormonal and miscellaneous side-effects of antipsychotic drugs. The questionnaire also includes 10 'red herring' items designed to detect service users who are incorrectly reporting adverse effects. Each item is rated on a 0–4 scale ranging from 'not at all' to 'very much'. The tool has a high degree of clinical utility and service users are normally able to complete the scale in 10–20 minutes. In an evaluation of the LUNSERS, Day et al. (1995) demonstrated that it had a high degree of validity and reliability.

Management

Helping service users to manage the side-effects of antipsychotic medication may improve satisfaction with treatment and increase compliance. It is therefore a crucial part of managing crisis and risk. Some of the most frequently observed and distressing side-effects of antipsychotic medication are outlined below, along with strategies for managing them.

- EPS may contribute significantly to non-compliance. Therefore they should be avoided or minimized as far as possible by lowering the dose of the neuroleptic, using adjunctive anticholinergics or switching to an alternative antipsychotic with a better EPS profile.

- Anticholinergic effects (such as blurred vision, dry mouth, constipation and urinary retention) can be managed using a number of simple measures which can easily be taught to service users. These include sipping water, chewing gum or using artificial saliva for dry mouth; using artificial tears for dry eyes; high-fibre diets, fibre supplements and increasing fluid intake for constipation.

- Whilst sedation is useful if service users are acutely ill or agitated it is an undesirable effect for those who have recovered from an acute episode. This is particularly problematic with chlorpromazine and clozapine.

- Some service users may experience a change in weight (usually an increase) when taking antipsychotic medication. This side-effect may lead to non-compliance and can also affect a service user's physical health because of the increased risk of cardiovascular problems. Service users' weight should be monitored regularly and any weight gain addressed promptly, for example by nutritional advice and implementation of an exercise programme.

INTERVENTIONS TO ENHANCE COMPLIANCE

A number of studies have evaluated the use of interventions to increase compliance. These include service user education (Gray & Smedley, 1996; Macpherson *et al.*, 1996; Smith *et al.*, 1992), behavioural tailoring (Boczkowski *et al.*, 1985) and compliance therapy (Kemp *et al.*, 1996).

In a randomized controlled trial of education about drug treatment by Macpherson and colleagues (1996), 64 service users with DSM IIIR schizophrenia were randomly assigned to receive either:

- one session of education about medication;
- three sessions of education about medication; or
- standard care.

The educational sessions were based on a specially designed booklet, drawn from psychoeducation literature and principles of general health education. Sessions lasted between 25 and 35 minutes. Techniques included rehearsal of material with questions and feedback.

A range of measures were used, including the Knowledge about Medication Questionnaire (KMQ) a tool designed to gauge service users' knowledge of antipsychotic treatment. Service users were assessed at baseline, immediately postintervention and at one month follow-up. Preintervention service users howed a poor understanding of their treatment. Both one and three sessions of ducation led to improvements in understanding about medication compared to tandard care. However, three sessions led to significantly greater knowledge gain han one session.

Smith *et al.* (1992) and Gray & Smedley (1996) also examined the effects of ducational interventions on knowledge about medication, insight into illness and ttitudes towards treatment. Smith *et al.* (1992) divided their intervention into our sessions, each session designed to cover a different aspect of schizophrenia. ession 1 examined the concept of schizophrenia, including possible causes and utcome. Session 2 focused on the symptoms of schizophrenia; session 3 mphasized the advantages, limitations, and side-effects of the treatment of chizophrenia; and session 4 outlined basic symptom management strategies. 'wenty-eight service users participated in the study and significant gains in their nowledge of treatment were observed postintervention. However, no significant hanges in insight or compliance with medication scores were reported.

Gray & Smedley (1996) examined the effects of education about medication n service users who were taking clozapine. Fifty service users were randomly ssigned to receive either three sessions of education or standard care. As in the mith *et al.* (1992) study, sessions focused on the concept, the symptoms and the reatment of schizophrenia. Service users' knowledge of the potential side-effects f medication increased and marginal improvements in insight were reported. lowever, no changes in service users' attitudes towards treatment, the measure nost predictive of compliance, were reported.

Boczkowski *et al.* (1985) took a very different approach to trying to improve ompliance. They assigned 36 male service users with chronic schizophrenia to eceive one session of either behavioural tailoring, service user education or a ontrol intervention. Behavioural tailoring involved informing service users of the mportance of complying with their medication and helping the service user to ailor their prescribed regimen so that it was better suited to their personal habits nd routines. Compliance was measured via pill counts at three time points: reintervention, one-month follow-up and three-month follow-up. Results uggested that service users who received behavioural tailoring were more ompliant following treatment than were the other groups.

In a seminal study, Kemp *et al.* (1996) evaluated the effectiveness of ompliance therapy (CT), a new intervention to enhance compliance in psychotic ervice users. Compliance therapy is a pragmatic intervention based on notivational interviewing and aims to help service users work through mbivalence about behaviour change. Key skills include the use of inductive juestioning, reflective listening, use of summarizing, investigating the pros and :ons of alternative courses of action and homing in on and reinforcing adaptive ttitudes and behaviours (Kemp *et al.*, 1997). CT is divided into three distinct »hases: phase 1 is concerned with reviewing the service user's illness history, phase ! explores ambivalence towards treatment and phase 3 highlights the need for reatment maintenance.

In the evaluation of CT, 47 service users were randomly assigned to receive 4–

6 sessions lasting 10–60 minutes each, of either CT or non-specific counselling. Service users were assessed preintervention, postintervention and at one, three and six-month follow-up using measures of insight into illness, attitudes toward treatment and compliance. Service users who received compliance therapy showed significantly greater improvements in attitudes towards treatment insight and compliance, which were sustained at six-month follow-up.

Interventions that address factors known to affect compliance, such as antipsychotic side-effects, attitudes towards treatment and insight have been repeatedly shown to be effective in improving compliance. Improved compliance through the use of medication management techniques will help minimize psychiatric risk. However, when crises do arise it may be necessary to resort to pharmacological interventions to control acutely disturbed service users. Mental health nurses will not only administer these drugs but will often be called upon to give advice about what drugs to prescribe.

THE ROLE OF PHARMACOLOGY IN THE MANAGEMENT OF VIOLENCE

A number of studies have examined the efficacy of rapid tranquillization, i.e. giving a psychotropic drug to control behavioural disturbances (Allan *et al.*, 1996; Dubin *et al.*, 1985; Dubin & Weis, 1986; Lenox *et al.*, 1992; Pilowsky *et al.* 1992; Resnick & Bunton, 1984; Salzman *et al.*, 1991; Tuason, 1986).

Pilowsky *et al.* (1992) surveyed the use of emergency prescribing in a general psychiatric hospital. One hundred and two incidents involving 60 service users were retrospectively examined. Injury to people or damage to property was fairly minor in 62% of incidents. However, more serious damage, including breaking furniture or smashing windows, was recorded in a third of incidents. The most commonly administered drugs were diazepam, haloperidol, chlorpromazine, droperidol, paraldehyde, amytal, lorazepam and nitrazepam. Fifty-two percent of drugs administered were given via an intramuscular injection and 48% were administered orally. In 41% of incidents a second drug was given.

The Royal College of Psychiatrists has recently published clinical practice guidelines on the management of violence. The review of the safety and efficacy of medication in the management of violence was systematic. The vast majority of research deals with the safety and efficacy of different agents in the treatment of difficult, disturbed, agitated or aggressive behaviour. They recommend that:

> ...*if rapid tranquillization is indicated because psychosocial methods of intervention have failed or are insufficient or inappropriate, benzodiazepines alone, or combined with an antipsychotic if a 'treatment' effect is also required, can be used with a reasonable degree of safety for managing violent behaviour.*

> (Royal College of Psychiatrists [RCP], 1997)

Significantly, the review found no evidence that a combination of several medications (polypharmacy) or the use of doses in excess of those recommended in the BNF produces better results (RCP, 1997).

Perhaps the most useful guidance on the management of acutely disturbed service users is found in the Maudsley Prescribing Guidelines, available directly from the Maudsley Hospital (Taylor et al., 1997). The algorithm for rapid control of acutely disturbed service users within these guidelines suggests that the first interventions used should be non-pharmacological (i.e. talking the service user down, distraction and seclusion). These psychological interventions may be augmented with the use of oral medication. If these interventions are not effective, 5–10 mg of haloperidol and 10 mg of diazepam (both administered orally) or 5–10 mg of droperidol and 2 mg of lorazepam (both administered via an intramuscular injection) should be considered. Following the administration of either of these combinations of drugs, the service user's respiratory rate and pulse and blood pressure should be closely monitored. If there is no response after 30 minutes then this should be repeated. If there is still no response, advice should be sought from a consultant or senior colleague.

CONCLUSION

A mental health crisis often results from poor medication management. This chapter has highlighted that non-compliance with medication is one of the primary reasons why psychotic service users relapse and require emergency admission to hospital. A number of factors associated with treatment non-compliance have been examined. Interventions that target these risk factors, for example minimizing side-effects or increasing the service user's understanding of treatment, may dramatically improve compliance and thus avoid crisis situations arising. However, service users may become violent and pharmacological interventions are often used to manage such situations. The recent Royal College of Psychiatrists guidelines demonstrate that the evidence base for rapid tranquillization is very poor and the guidelines which are proposed are tentative.

REFERENCES

Adler, L.A., Anrist, N., Reiter, S. & Rotrosen, J. (1989) Neuroleptic-induced akathisia: a review. *Psychopharmacology*. 97, 1–11.

Allan, E.R., Alpert, M.A., Sison, C.E. *et al.* (1996) Adjunctive nadolol in the treatment of acutely aggressive schizophrenic patients. *Journal of Clinical Psychiatry*. 57:10, 455–459.

Angermeyer, M.C. & Matschinger, H. (1994) Lay beliefs about schizophrenic disorder: the results of a population survey in Germany. Lubeck symposium: The role of compliance in the treatment of schizophrenia. *Acta Psychiatrica Scandinavica*. 89 (supplement 382), 39–45.

Appelbaum, P.S. & Gutheil, T.G. (1980) Drug refusal: a study of psychiatric inpatients. *American Journal of Psychiatry*. 137, 340–346.

Babiker, I.E. (1986) Noncompliance in schizophrenia. *Psychiatric Developments*. 4, 329–337.

Barnes, T.R.E. (1989) A rating scale for drug-induced akathisia. *British Journal of Psychiatry*. 154, 672–676.

Bartko, G., Herceg, I. & Zador, G. (1988) Clinical symptomatology and drug compliance in schizophrenic patients. *Acta Psychiatrica Scandinavica*. 77, 74–76.

Bennett, J., Done, J. & Hunt, B. (1991) Drugs and the CPN. *Nursing Times*. 44, 38–40.

Bennett, J., Done, J. & Hunt, B. (1995a) Assessing the side effects of antipsychotic drugs: a survey of CPN practice. *Journal of Psychiatric and Mental Health Nursing*. 2:3, 177–182.

Bennett, J., Done, J., Harrison-Read, P. & Hunt, B. (1995b) Development of a rating scale/checklist to assess the side effects of antipsychotics by community psychiatric nurses. In: C. Brooker & E. White (eds) *Community Psychiatric Nursing: A Research Perspective*, Volume 3. London: Chapman & Hall, pp.1–19.

Boczkowski, J.A., Zeichner, A. & DeSanto, N. (1985) Neuroleptic compliance among chronic schizophrenic outpatients: an intervention outcome report. *Journal of Consulting and Clinical Psychology*. 53, 666–671.

Buchanan, A. (1992) A two-year prospective study of treatment compliance in patients with schizophrenia. *Psychological Medicine*. 22, 787–797.

Chaplin, R. & McGuigan, S. (1996) Antipsychotic dose: from research to clinical practice. *Psychiatric Bulletin*. 20, 452–454.

Chouinard, G., Ross-Chouinard, A., Annable, L. & Jones, B.D. (1980) Extrapyramidal rating scale. *Canadian Journal of Neurological Sciences*. 7, 233.

Clozapine Study Group (1993) The safety and efficacy of clozapine in severe treatment-resistant schizophrenic patients in the UK. *British Journal of Psychiatry*. 163, 150–154.

Cornwall, P.L., Hassanyeh, F. & Horn, C. (1996) High-dose antipsychotic medication. *Psychiatric Bulletin*. 20, 676–680.

Day, J., Wood, G., Dewey, M. & Bentall, R.P. (1995) A self-rating scale for measuring neuroleptic side-effects: validation in a group of schizophrenic patients. *British Journal of Psychiatry*. 166, 650–653.

Dubin, W.R. & Weis, K.J. (1986) Rapid tranquillisation: a comparison of thiothixene with loxapine. *Journal of Clinical Psychiatry*. 47:6, 294–297.

Dubin, W.R., Waxman, H.M., Weiss, K.J., Ramchandani, D. & Tavani-Petrone, C. (1985) Rapid tranquillisation: the efficacy of oral concentrate. *Journal of Clinical Psychiatry*. 46:11, 475–478.

Fleischhaker, W., Bergmann, K.J., Perovich, R. *et al.* (1989) The Hillside akathisia scale: a new rating instrument for neuroleptic-induced akathisia, parkinsonism and hyperkinesia. *Psychopharmacological Bulletin*. 25:2, 222–226.

Geller, J.L. (1982) State hospital patients and their medication: do they know what they take? *American Journal of Psychiatry*. 139:5, 611–615.

Gray, R. & Gournay, K. (1997) Medication management in psychotic disorders: A systematic review of nursing research. London: Institute of Psychiatry, unpublished report.

Gray, R. & Smedley, N. (1996) A controlled trial of educational interventions in people with schizophrenia. Presented at the First Psychotic Episodes of Schizophrenia Conference, Amsterdam, Netherlands, 28–29 November.

Gray, R., Gournay, K. & Taylor, D. (1997) New drug treatments in schizophrenia: implications for mental health nurses. *Mental Health Practice*. 1:1, 20–23.

Green, J.H. (1988) Frequent rehospitalization and non-compliance with treatment. *Hospital and Community Psychiatry*. 39, 963–966.

Guy, W. (1976) *ECDEU Assessment Manual for Psychopharmacology*, Revised edn. Washington: US Department of Health Education and Welfare.

Haase, H.J. (1954) Ubervorkommen und Deutung des psychomotorischen Parkinsonsyndroms bei Megaphen-bzw. *Largactil-Dauerbehandlung*. Nervenartzt, 25, 486.

Haase, H.J. (1978) The purely neuroleptic effect and its relation to the 'neuroleptic threshold'. *Acta Psychiatrica Belgica*. 78, 19–36.

Hayward, P., Chan, N., Kemp, R., Youle, S. & David, A. (1995) Medication self-management: a preliminary report on an intervention to improve medication compliance. *Journal of Mental Health*. 4:5, 511–519.

Hillam, J. & Evans, C. (1996) Neuroleptic drug use in psychiatric intensive therapy units: problems with complying with the consensus statement. *Psychiatric Bulletin*. 20, 82–84.

Hoge, S.K., Appelbaum, P.S., Lawlor, T. *et al.* (1990) A prospective, multi-centre study of patients' refusal of antipsychotic medication. *Archives of General Psychiatry*. 47:10, 949–956.

Kane, M.D., Honigfeld, G., Singer, J. & Meltzer, H. (1988) Clozapine for the treatment-resistant schizophrenic. *Archives of General Psychiatry*. 45:9, 789–796.

Kemp, R. & David, A. (1995) Insight and adherence to treatment in psychotic disorders. *British Journal of Hospital Medicine*. 54, 222–227.

Kemp, R., Hayward, P., Applewhaite, G., Everitt, B. & David, A. (1996) Compliance therapy in psychotic patients: a randomised controlled trial. *British Medical Journal*. 312, 345–349.

Kemp, R., Hayward, P. & David, A. (1997) *Compliance Therapy Manual*. London: Bethlem and Maudsley NHS Trust.

Kissling, W, (1994) Compliance, quality assurance and standards for relapse prevention in schizophrenia. *Acta Psychiatrica Scandinavica*. 89 (supplement 382), 16–24.

Krasuck, C. & MacFarlane, F. (1996) Electrocardiograms, high-dose antipsychotic treatment and College guidelines. *Psychiatric Bulletin*. 20, 326–330

Lane, R.D., Glazer, W.M., Hansen, T.E., Berman, W.H. & Kramer, S.I. (1985) Assessment of tardive dyskinesia using the Abnormal Involuntary Movements Scale. *Journal of Nervous and Mental Disorders*. 173:6, 353–357.

Lenox, R.H., Newhouse, P.A., Creelman, W.L. & Whitaker, T.M. (1992) Adjunctive treatment of manic agitation with lorazepam versus haloperidol: a double-blind study. *Journal of Clinical Psychiatry*. 53:2, 47–52.

Lin, H.F., Spiga, R. & Fortsch, W. (1979) Insight and adherence to medication in chronic schizophrenics. *Journal of Clinical Psychiatry*. 40, 430–432.

Lingjaerde, O., Ahlfors, U.G., Bech, P., Dencker, S.J. & Elgen, K. (1987) The UKU side effects rating scale. *Acta Psychiatrica Scandinavica*. 76 (supplement 334), 83–94.

Macpherson, R., Jerrom, B. & Hughes, A. (1996) A controlled study of education and drug treatment in schizophrenia. *British Journal of Psychiatry*. 168, 709–717.

Marder, S.R., Mebane, A., Chien, C. *et al.* (1983) A comparison of patients who refuse and consent to neuroleptic treatment. *American Journal of Psychiatry*. 140:4, 470–472.

Matted, J.A (1989) Clozapine for refractory schizophrenia: an open study of 14 patients treated for up to two years. *Journal of Clinical Psychiatry*. 50, 389–391.

McEvoy, J.P., Freter, S., Everett, G. et al. (1989) Insight and the clinical outcome of schizophrenic patients. *Journal of Nervous and Mental Disorders*. 177:1, 48–51.

Meltzer, H.Y., Matsubara, S. & Lee, J.C. (1989) Classification of typical and atypical antipsychotic drugs on the basis of D1 and D2 and serotonin 2 pKi values. *Journal of Pharmacology and Experimental Therapeutics*. 251, 238–246.

Michaux, W.W. (1961) Side effects, resistance and dosage deviations in psychiatric outpatients treated with tranquillisers. *Journal of Nervous and Mental Disease*. 133, 203–212.

Mindham, R.H.S. (1976) Assessment of drug-induced extrapyramidal reactions and of drug given for their control. *British Journal of Clinical Pharmacology*. 3 (supplement), 395–400.

Munetz, M. & Benjamine, S. (1988) How to examine patients using the Abnormal Involuntary Movements Scale. *Hospital and Community Psychiatry*. 39, 1172–1177.

Nelson, A. (1975) Drug default among schizophrenic patients. *American Journal of Hospital Pharmacy*. 32, 1237–1242.

Newton, K.L., Murthy, R. & Qureshi, J. (1996) Antipsychotic prescribing in light of the consensus statement of the College. *Psychiatric Bulletin*. 21, 408–410.

Owen, R.R., Beake, B.J., Marby, D., Dessain, E.C. & Cole, J.O. (1989) Response to clozapine in chronic psychotic patients. *Psychopharmacological Bulletin*. 25:2, 253–256.

Pilowsky, L.S., Ring, P.J., Battersby, M. & Lader, M. (1992) Rapid tranquillisation. A survey of emergency prescribing in a general psychiatric hospital. *British Journal of Psychiatry*. 160, 831–835.

Resnick, M. & Bunton, B.T. (1984) Droperidol vs. haloperidol in the initial management of acutely agitated patients. *Journal of Clinical Psychiatry*. 45:7, 298–299.

Richelson, E. (1984) Neuroleptic affinities for human brain receptors and their use in predicting adverse effects. *Journal of Clinical Psychiatry*. 45:7, 331–336.

Royal College of Psychiatrists (1997) *The Management of Violence in Clinical Settings: An Evidence Based Guideline*. London: RCP's Clinical Practice Guidelines Programme.

Salzman, C., Solomon, D., Miyawaki, E. et al. (1991) Parenteral lorazepam versus parenteral haloperidol for the control of psychotic disruptive behaviour. *Journal of Clinical Psychiatry*. 52:4, 177–180.

Seeman, P. (1980) Brain dopamine receptors. *Pharmacological Review*. 32, 229–313.

Simpson, G.M. & Angus, J.W.S. (1970) A rating scale for extrapyramidal side effects. *Acta Psychiatrica Scandinivica*. 212 (supplement 44), 11–19.

Simpson, G.M., Lee, J.H., Zoubok, B. & Gardos, G. (1979) A rating scale for tardive dyskinesia. *Psychopharmacology*. 64, 171–179.

Smith, J., Birchwood, M. & Haddrell, A. (1992) Informing people with schizophrenia about their illness: the effect on residual symptoms. *Journal of Mental Health*. 1, 61–70.

Taylor, D., Duncan, D., McConnell, H. & Abel, K. (1997) *Prescribing Guidelines*, 4th ed. London: Bethlem and Maudsley NHS Trust.

Torrey, E.T. (1994) Violent behaviour by individuals with serious mental illness. Special issue: Violent behaviour and mental illness. *Hospital and Community Psychiatry*. 45:7, 653–662.

Tuason, V.B. (1986) A comparison of parenteral loxapine and haloperidol in hostile and aggressive acutely schizophrenic patients. *Journal of Clinical Psychiatry*. 47:3, 126–129.

van Putten, T. (1974) Why do schizophrenic patients refuse to take their drugs? *Archives of General Psychiatry.* 31, 67–72.

van Putten, T. & Marder, S.R. (1986) Towards a more reliable diagnosis of akathisia. *Archives of General Psychiatry.* 43, 1015–1016.

van Putten, T. & Marder, S.R. (1987) Behavioural toxicity of antipsychotic drugs. *Journal of Clinical Psychiatry.* 48 (supplement 9), 13–19.

van Putten, T., Crumpton, E. & Yale, C. (1976) Drug refusal in schizophrenia and the wish to be crazy. *Archives of General Psychiatry.* 33, 1443–1446.

van Putten, T., May, P.R., Marder, S.R. & Wittman, L.A. (1981) Subjective response to antipsychotic drugs. *Archives of General Psychiatry.* 38, 187–190.

van Wielinck, P.S. & Leysen, J.E. (1983) Choice of neuroleptics based on in vitro pharmacology. *Journal of Drug Research.* 8, 1984–1997.

Weiden, P.J., Shaw, E. & Mann, J. (1986) Causes of neuroleptic non-compliance. *Psychiatry Annals.* 16, 571–575.

Wojckik, J., Glenberg, A., La Brie, R.A. & Mieske, M. (1980) Prevalence of tardive dyskinesia in an outpatient population. *Comprehensive Psychiatry.* 21, 370–379.

Yorston, G. & Pinney, A. (1997) Use of high dose antipsychotic medication. *Psychiatric Bulletin.* 21, 566–569.

Young, J.L., Zonana, H.V. & Shepler, L.S. (1986) Medication non-compliance in schizophrenia: codification and update. *Bulletin of the American Academy of Psychiatry and Law.* 14:2, 105–122.

13 ISSUES IN CLINICAL AND ACTUARIAL ASSESSMENT OF CRISIS AND RISK

Barry Thirkettle and Tony Ryan

INTRODUCTION

Within current practice, mental health nurses and other professionals are expected to manage risks and crises associated with people who have mental health needs. This has arisen for a number of reasons, such as public concern about people with mental health problems receiving community care, the proximity of mental health nurses to service users in both hospital and community settings, the professionalization of nursing, the trend towards evidence-based practice and an increasing awareness of the implications for service users and others when risk assessments prove to be wrong.

Risk prediction, or risk assessment, forms a key part in the management of risk. It is not an exact science since attempting to forecast what a person might do in the future, irrespective of the state of their mental health, is subject to the idiosyncrasies of human nature and a combination of many not always identifiable or predictable variables which may be specific to the individual situation. Nevertheless, risk assessment is a fundamental part of the role of mental health nurses and consequently an awareness of the accuracy and limitations of such forecasting and the factors that influence this are essential if mental health nursing practice is to develop in this area.

MENTAL HEALTH RISKS AND RISK FACTORS

Although risk can be seen as a balance between potentially negative and potentially positive outcomes, within the context of mental health care the term 'risk' is mainly used to express the likelihood of an adverse or harmful event occurring. People with mental health problems are perceived to face a number of risks including being vulnerable, disempowered or dependent on others (Ryan, 1998). They are also at a high risk of being imprisoned, becoming homeless or being stigmatized (see Ryan, 1996, for a review). Naturally, it is important that mental health nurses assess all forms of risk relating to those with whom they work. However, this chapter will concentrate on the areas of risk which are currently given prominence by mental health professionals, policymakers and risk managers (Department of Health, 1996; Tan & McDonough, 1990). These areas are risk of violence to others, risk of self-harm (including parasuicide, i.e. attempted suicide), risk of suicide and risk of serious self-neglect. Although the chapter will focus specifically on these areas of risk, the principles and issues discussed will be relevant to the many other areas of risk associated with caring for people with a mental health problem.

When attempting to make a risk prediction, it is essential to know the factors which appear to correlate with a particular type of harmful behaviour and which are therefore associated with an increased likelihood of a particular risk occurring. The risk factors associated with the areas of risk under discussion are listed in Boxes 13.1–3. Although the presence or absence of particular factors does not guarantee the accuracy of any risk prediction, they provide a position from which to start. For example, in an assessment of violence, the risk associated with a 20-year-old single man who misuses alcohol and has a diagnosis of paranoid schizophrenia will be greater than the risk associated with a 45-year-old mother

---

Box 13.1

Risk factors associated with violence to others

Demographic factors
- Youth
- Male
- Low socioeconomic status
- Unstable living arrangements
- Unstable or no employment

Clinical factors
- Alcohol or drug misuse
- Paranoid psychosis
- Manic depression
- Schizophrenia
- Psychotic depression
- Active psychotic symptoms

Other factors
- Impassivity
- Anger
- Previous history of violence
- Non-compliance with medication
- Loss of family support
- Deterioration in personal relationships
- Declared violent intentions and attitudes
- Loss of contact

(Adapted from Alberg *et al.*, 1996; Lipsedge, 1995; Monahan, 1992)

Box 13.2
Risk factors associated with deliberate self-harm and suicide

Demographic factors
- Older men (suicide)
- Men in late teens or early 20s (suicide)
- Women (self-harm)
- People under 30 years (self-harm)
- Divorced, widowed or single

Clinical factors
- Depression
- Schizophrenia
- Chronic sleep disorders
- Alcohol or drug misuse
- Cognitive dysfunction
- Personality disorder
- Pessimism
- Family history of mood disorder, suicide or alcoholism
- Signs of self-neglect

Other factors
- Declared suicidal or self-harm intent
- Preparation behaviour, e.g. hoarding tablets
- History of deliberate self-harm, particularly in the previous six months
- Lethality of previous attempts
- Isolation
- Unemployed or retired
- Recent adverse life events
- Chronic pain and terminal illness
- Post trauma
- Stressful living conditions

(Adapted from Alberg *et al.*, 1996; Duffy, 1993; Hughes & Owen, 1996; Lipsedge, 1995; Williams & Morgan, 1994)

Box 13.3

Risk factors associated with self-neglect

Demographic factors
- Elderly people (especially men)
- Low intelligence

Clinical factors
- Schizophrenia
- Depression
- Mania
- Alcohol or drug misuse
- Dementia
- Confusional states

Other factors
- Poor management of mental health
- Post trauma

(Adapted from Alberg *et al.*, 1996)

---

with a depressive illness who does not drink or take drugs. Whilst it is always possible that the woman may be violent and the man not, the factors for violence are more closely associated with the profile of the man than the woman.

One point that emerges from Boxes 13.1–3 is that having a mental illness appears to be a risk factor for all the different types of risk under discussion. Most people who commit suicide have some form of mental illness, most commonly depression, schizophrenia or alcohol dependency (Hawton, 1987; King, 1994). A number of studies have also shown that there is an association between some people who experience a mental illness, particularly schizophrenia, and violent behaviour (Humphreys *et al.*, 1992; Lindqvist & Allebeck, 1990; Link *et al.*, 1992; Link & Stueve, 1994; Mullen, 1997; Nobel & Rodger, 1989; Swanson, 1994; Taylor, 1985). However, this association has only recently been generally accepted by most researchers and clinicians. This is in part due to the lack of clarity about which factors contribute most to violence; for example, schizophrenia or alcohol misuse. John Monahan was one of the leading advocates for the view that there is no relationship between mental illness and violence (see Monahan, 1981). However, the following passage reflects how his view has changed.

On the one hand, the general public and their elected representatives appear firmly committed to the view that mental disorder and violence are connected.

> *On the other hand many social science researchers and the patient advocates*
> *who cite them seem equally convinced that no such connection exists. Although*
> *I have long been in the latter camp, I now believe that there may be a*
> *relationship between mental disorder and violent behaviour, one that cannot be*
> *fobbed off as chance or explained away by other factors that may cause them*
> *both.*
>
> (Monahan, 1992, p.511)

However, although there definitely does appear to be some form of relationship between having a mental illness and being violent, it is important to note that in *absolute* terms the risk of violence-associated mental illness is still very low. Other factors such as low social class, young age, male gender and substance and alcohol abuse are much better predictors of violence than mental state (Pilgrim & Rogers, 1996). With respect to suicide the situation is similar; the absolute number of suicides is very small and the factors associated with it lack specificity. As we will see later in this chapter, this makes it difficult to develop tools with high predictive value for suicides. It is easier to predict higher frequency events such as self-harm and parasuicide.

The most robust clinical predictor of future suicidal behaviour is a history of self-harm or suicidal behaviour (Lipsedge, 1995). Up to 40% of people who eventually commit suicide have made a prior suicide attempt and there is a 32% increase in relative risk associated with each prior attempt (Malone *et al.*, 1995). Identification of depressed people with a history of suicidal behaviour is essential for the detection of people at high risk of suicide. Hopelessness and pessimism have also been found to be important factors related to suicidal ideation and intent and are better as predictors of suicide than depression *per se* (Beck & Weishaar, 1990). However, hopelessness and pessimism appear to be less reliable predictors of future parasuicidal behaviour (Hughes & Neimeyer, 1993). The lethality of previous suicide attempts is also positively correlated with future risk, but only if the person has a reasonably accurate knowledge of the probable lethality of the chosen means (Beck & Weishaar, 1990). This means that one must be cautious of misinterpreting a non-lethal attempt as simply being a gesture, as it may be that the person definitely wanted to die but, without realizing it, had chosen an ineffective means.

Relatively little research has been published on risk assessment for self-neglect and the factors associated with it. However, two useful reviews of the self-neglect concept are provided by Reed & Leonard (1989) and Johnson & Adams (1996). Comparing the risk factors in Box 13.2 and in Box 13.3, it can be seen that there is considerable overlap between the risk factors for suicide and self-harm and those for self-neglect. In fact, signs of self-neglect have been identified as a risk factor for suicide and self-harm. It is also arguable that in instances where the self-neglect is deliberate rather than by omission, it could be classified as a type of deliberate self-harm.

It is worth noting that some risk factors present in the general population appear to have a different weighting as far as people with mental illness are oncerned. For example, Appleby (1997) points out with respect to suicide risk hat mental illness is such a powerful risk factor that it can obliterate the effect of other variables. Mullen (1997) also points out that although crimes of violence among people without a mental illness are almost exclusively a male preserve, this disparity is far less marked among those with mental health needs. Furthermore, women with schizophrenia appear to have a much higher risk for violence than women with other mental illnesses (Lindqvist & Allebeck, 1990; Wessely, 1997).

Risk factors such as those shown in Boxes 13.1–3 are generally more effective as predictors of risk in the longer term rather than in the more immediate future. This is not surprising as a longer time period provides a greater opportunity for the risk behaviour to occur. Other temporal factors also appear to be relevant, particularly in relation to suicide risk. Suicide risk appears to increase during the period immediately after the admission and in the first few weeks following discharge and during weekend leave (Goldcare et al., 1993; Morgan & Priest, 1991). Goldcare et al. (1993) also showed that shorter lengths of stay appeared to lead to an increased risk of suicide in some people. Morgan (1997) suggests reasons why there appears to be an increased risk when the clinical state appears to be improving. In a small number of cases, the improvement is a false one as the final decision to go ahead with the suicide can lead to an outwardly deceptive calm. Morgan also highlights the real but misleading improvement produced by the protective effects of the hospital admission, which disappear once the person is discharged.

One can see from Boxes 13.1–3 that some factors appear to be permanent and unchangeable, whereas others can change with time. Limandri & Sheridan (1995) differentiate between static and dynamic predictors. Static predictors are demographic factors that cannot be altered, such as gender, age and previous history, while the dynamic factors include attitudes, symptoms and behaviours that can be manipulated to reduce risk through various interventions. Mental illness in itself can be seen as a dynamic risk factor given that in many cases it will be associated with particular symptomatologies, behaviours and attitudes that may increase the likelihood of violence to self or others. Conversely, when the symptoms are controlled, the risk may be much less. Several studies have also shown that the risk of violence is greater if active psychotic symptoms are present, particularly delusional beliefs and passivity experiences (Addad et al., 1988; Krakowski-Jaeger & Volavka, 1988; Taylor, 1985). This means that if these symptoms are identified during the risk assessment process and steps can be taken to control them, the risk of violence will be reduced.

PREDICTING RISK

Within mental health care, the aim of a risk assessment is to separate those people who have a high probability of coming to harm or harming others from those people where this probability is low. Box 13.4 illustrates the possible outcomes when making a risk assessment. A risk assessment that correctly identifies all or most of the people at high risk, that is *true positives*, is said to have a high level of

Box 13.4

Outcomes of risk prediction

True positive Correctly predicting that an event will occur	True negative Correctly predicting that an event will not occur
False positive Predicting an event that does not occur	False negative Predicting an event will not take place that subsequently occurs

sensitivity. However, if the risk assessment incorrectly identifies several people as falling within the high-risk group when really they are a low risk, that is *false positives*, then the risk assessment is said to have a low level of *specificity*. A good risk assessment has a high level of both sensitivity and specificity.

The consequences of inaccurate risk assessment can be extremely serious for those involved. For example, in the case of a risk assessment of violence that proves to be a *false-negative* prediction, there are two immediate consequences: the injuries that occur to the victim of the violence and the sanctions placed upon the assailant. A further consequence, which is often ignored, can be guilty feelings of those who made the false negative prediction as they have to live with the consequences and the knowledge that their prediction was wrong. The consequences of false positives can also be significant for the service user. To predict that a service user may be dangerous to themselves or other people when they are not can lead to unnecessary treatments being given. Such predictions can also lead to unjustifiable supervision or detention of service users. These concerns have led some commentators to suggest that attempts to predict violence and other forms of risk might create more problems than solutions (Miller & Morris, 1988).

Vinestock (1996) points out that although risk assessment will not enable the clinician to make 100% accurate decisions and to avoid all risk, it does help to make defensible decisions – defensible clinically, logically and medicolegally. Vinestock suggests that the purpose of any risk assessment is to achieve the best possible grasp of the likely behaviour of a person and to elicit sufficient detail for risk factors to be minimized and appropriately managed. One important principle is that the effort and investment in predicting risk must justify returns.

TYPES OF RISK ASSESSMENT

There are two forms of assessing risk in mental health today that may be used separately or in combination; these are clinical risk assessment and actuarial risk assessment. Clinical risk assessment normally involves using a semistructured format to interview the person and others of significance such as relatives, carers, friends and professionals from other agencies who may have had contact with the person. Clinical risk assessment can also be enhanced through observations of the person and a thorough reading of their clinical records. Clinical records can reveal a history of previous risk behaviour, therefore it is essential for incidents to be documented in detail to support future risk assessments. Clinical risk assessment depends heavily on the clinical judgement, experience and knowledge of the individual person. By contrast, actuarial assessments match individuals with population-based indicators or risk factors in a very structured framework, using instruments which have been based on actuarial or statistical data.

MODELS OF CLINICAL RISK ASSESSMENT

Limandri & Sheridan (1995) suggest that according to the current literature, there are three models of clinical prediction. The *linear model* can be ideally suited to forensic environments where there are significant legal implications for all involved since the logic of the approach can easily be understood in the courtroom. Linear models typically follow a series of steps; for example, in the case of violence: clarifying the risk, assessing its deadliness, identifying any specific intended victims, identifying the immediacy of the risk and taking account of the relationship between assailant and intended victim. These steps are then followed by a decision on the most appropriate method of managing the threat whether in hospital, under detention or voluntarily, or in the community. The main drawback is that for it to work logically, or objectively, contextual factors are largely ignored. In essence, the method can become more important than the content.

The *hypothetic-inductive model* relies more on the nurse's previous experience while looking for patterns of behaviour and particular cues to the risk behaviour, such as impulsivity or trauma. A constant comparison between theoretical notions and the specific context of the case provides the path towards decision making. As a the hypothetical assumption, is tested against previous experience and existing being assessed and others previously assessed be limited by the nurse's previous experience and preferred methods of intervention. Consequently, it is least effective

The final method is the ris whether it is the risk of violence, self- being less dichotomous – not simply stating will occur. Instead, the nurse should assume that some are more possible than others. Personal r service user are identified and then placed into the can then rate the likelihood of each outcome given the contexts that may be available for the service user. This is don the identified risks with perceived benefits. A decision is then made on the l of the ratings that have been calculated and an appropriate timescale. The principal drawback with this method is that it can be time consuming, leaving the nurse weighed down by all the possibilities, particularly given that outcomes are potentially infinite.

CRITICISMS OF CLINICAL RISK ASSESSMENT

Clinical risk assessment has been criticized for being highly subjective and relying too heavily on qualitative data. Such assessments of risk can be subject to the biases of the person making the assessment, their previous experiences, their theoretical perspective and their preferred methods of intervention. Consequently, they can be prone to inconsistencies, not merely between assessors but by the same assessor over time. Carrying out clinical risk assessments on a multidisciplinary basis can in theory reduce such biases. However, it has been suggested that in the process of sharing information about potential risk between members of the multidisciplinary team, the group dynamic can in itself lead to biases. Whilst in theory multidisciplinary working should provide greater objectivity, strong team members, such as those with the greatest experience, can affect colleagues, whether they are aware of such influences or not. Clearly, all members of the multidisciplinary team, including nurses, need to be aware of such influences and ensure that the risk assessment takes into account the findings and views of all team members. Some studies have shown that clinicians working together achieve a greater level of accuracy in their predictions than those working alone (Holloway, 1997; Werner et al., 1990).

In the past, clinical assessment of risk of violence has been criticized for its poor accuracy (Litwack et al., 1993; Monahan, 1981, 1988; Quinsey & Maguire, 1979, 1986). Monahan (1981), examining the accuracy of clinical judgements predicting violent behaviour towards others, found that psychiatrists and psychologists were accurate in no more than one out of three predictions of violent behaviour among institutionalized populations. More recently, these criticisms have been questioned and challenged as these findings were biased by methodological issues (Monahan, 1988; Monahan & Steadman, 1994; Mossman, 1994).

A major methodological problem is that once a person has been identified as being potentially violent, it is more likely that preventive measures will be taken to minimize the risk of the violent behaviour occurring. These cases may thus appear as false positives, whereas without the intervention measures they may have been true positives. This makes it difficult to verify whether or not the prediction would have come true. Conversely, those who have been predicted as not likely to be violent are more likely to be discharged into the community and if they do in fact become violent, it is possible that this violent behaviour will not be detected or reported. Other difficulties include diagnostic groupings being too inclusive, lack of definition of what is classed as violent behaviour, individual situational variables not being identified or controlled for and the individual context not being taken into account.

In a rare community-based study, Lidz and colleagues (1993) overcame the problem of clinicians intervening once a person is identified as being more likely to be violent. They asked nurses and psychiatrists in a psychiatric emergency room of a large urban hospital to assess potential patient violence to others during a six-month period after assessment. They found that the accuracy of clinicians' predictions of male violence was significantly better than by chance, whereas the predictions for violence by women did not differ from chance. They concluded that clinicians can predict dangerousness at a better than chance level even when demographic factors are controlled, even though the relatively low sensitivity and specificity of their predictions showed that there is substantial room for improvement. This study supports the view that clinical judgement has been undervalued in previous research. Not only did the clinicians pick out a statistically more violent group, but the violence that the predicted group committed was more serious than the acts of the comparison group. The finding that clinicians had great difficulty predicting violence in women may reflect their poor understanding of the fact that having a mental illness appears to increase the likelihood of women being violent.

In another study of violent behaviour among psychiatric inpatients, McNeil & Binder (1991) found that although the overall rate of assaults was overpredicted, in the short term there was a close correspondence between nurses' and physicians' clinical estimates of people becoming violent and later displaying violence. Studies of people in the community are much rarer, with the one notable exception discussed above.

Problems have also been highlighted with regard to the clinical risk assessment of suicide and self-harm behaviour. Maltsberger & Rosenberg (1990) write that:

> Suicide risk assessment is fraught with difficulty, the confident prediction of suicide is impossible at present, clinicians are forced to make assessments as best they can, for there is no standard scientific method on which all agree, and according to which risk assessments can be made.
>
> (p.3)

Goldstein et al. (1991) developed a model based on a number of risk factors, including a history of prior suicide attempts, and found that out of 1906 depressed people, they were unable to identify any of the 46 people who actually committed suicide.

Hughes (1996) goes so far as to conclude that most scientific studies to date show that clinicians cannot predict individual suicide. Although the suicide rate for hospitalized psychiatric patients is much higher than for the general population, it is argued that it is still too low to make accurate risk predictions. Consequently, many studies have focused on other behaviours such as parasuicide and suicidal ideation (Hughes & Neimeyer, 1993), which occur at much higher frequency than completed suicide. Morgan (1997) puts forward a different view and suggests that the infrequency of suicides may in fact be an indication of how good GPs are at treating depression. If the risk assessment has been accurate and appropriate interventions have been taken, then the suicide or violent incident will not have occurred. Prediction of suicide is made difficult by it being a relatively infrequent event, even among high-risk groups.

Appleby (1997) suggests that there needs to be a balance between risk factor and protective factors, although at present we know little about the latter. A person with numerous risk factors may not be at high risk if each risk is counterbalanced. Similarly, a person who is stable may be at high risk if some of the protective factors are removed. This may explain the increased incidence of suicides immediately following discharge because the care received within the hospital has a protective effect. The clinical assessment of risk must also aim at an accurate appraisal of the relative weightings of the various risk factors in each individual case (Morgan, 1997).

Malone et al. (1995) found that clinicians failed to document adequately the presence of a lifetime history of suicide attempts, recent suicide ideation or planning behaviour. As has already been pointed out, it is very useful to maintain accurate and detailed records of any incidents as these data can be used to support clinical risk assessment at a later date and help to avoid any history of previous risk behaviour being overlooked.

Risk assessment is an ongoing process and risk factors change. Mullen (1997) concludes that in the short term clinicians' risk predictions would appear to be reasonably reliable, although risk assessments in the medium and long term are less reliable. Second, the accuracy of risk predictions appears to decline over time and moves from a success level that is greater than chance to one that is not (Gunn, 1993). Pokorny (1983), with respect to suicide risk assessment, points out that the clinician works in the timeframe of minutes, hours or days in dealing with the suicidal crisis, whereas the frame of months or years is used by clinical researchers. He questioned whether the clinician's problem is suicide prediction or more to do with identifying a suicidal crisis already underway. Nurses are the team members who in many instances have the most frequent contact with the individual service user. Therefore, they have an important role to play in monitoring changes in the person's situation, behaviour or mental state that may change their level of risk.

ACTUARIAL RISK ASSESSMENT

A number of risk assessment tools used to assess and predict risk of violence, suicide and self-harm can be identified from the literature. Examples of these tools are listed in Tables 13.1 and 13.2 respectively. Some of these tools, such as the Suicide Ideation Scale (SSI; Beck et al., 1979), were designed specifically to study the correlation of a specific risk factor with a specific risk behaviour, in this example suicide ideation and suicide. Other tools, such as the Nurses' Outcome Evaluation Scale (NOSIE; Honigfeld, 1976), are more general measures covering a number of variables and potential risk factors. NOSIE, for example, not only covers risk factors for violence but also risk factors for suicide and self-harm.

There appears to be little published research on the use of risk assessment tools for self-neglect. However, some more general measures which could be used to identify and quantify some of the risk factors associated with self-neglect could include the Brief Psychiatric Rating Scale (BPRS; Overall & Goreham, 1962) and the Mini Mental State Examination (MMSE; Folstein et al., 1975).

Table 13.1

Examples of risk assessment tools used to predict violence

Name of tool	Additional information	Reference
Anger Rating Index	Seven-item component of a larger 36-item scale	(Novaco, 1994)
Buss–Durkee Hostility Inventory	75-item scale composed of eight subscales covering physical assault, indirect hostility, irritability, negativism, resentment, suspicion, verbal hostility and guilt	(Buss & Durkee, 1957)
State-Trait Anger Expression Inventory (STAXI)		(Spielberger et al., 1988)
Novaco Provocation Inventory (NPI)	80-item self-report instrument in two parts	(Novaco, 1975)
Brief Anger Aggression Questionnaire (BAAQ)	Six-item scale	(Maiuro et al., 1987)
Barratt Impulsiveness Scale (BIS-11)	11th revision still undergoing further development	(Barratt, 1994)
Psychopathy Checklist – Revised (PCL-R)	20-item scale, screening version (PCL-SV), under development	(Hart et al., 1994)
Michigan Alcoholism Screening Test (MAST)		(Selzer, 1971)
Drug Abuse Screening Test (DAST)		(Skinner, 1982)
Psychiatric Epidemiology Research Interview (PERI)	Contains scales and measures of psychotic symptoms, violent behaviours and self-reported arrests	(Dohrenwend et al., 1986)
Nurses' Observation Scale for Inpatient Evaluation (NOSIE)	Contains several items concerning identifying active psychotic symptoms	(Honigfeld, 1976)
Brief Psychiatric Rating Scale (BPRS)	Contains 18 symptom scales	(Overall & Goreham, 1962)
Overt Aggression Scale	A behavioural checklist used by nurses	(Yudofsky et al., 1986)
Maudsley Assessment of Delusions Scale (MADS)	Available as brief and extended versions	(Taylor et al., 1994)

As with clinical risk assessment, a number of criticisms have been levelled at actuarial risk assessment. Most actuarial tools have been developed for research purposes rather than for clinical practice and so they do not always meet the needs of everyday situations as well as nurses and other clinicians would like. A study by Woods (1996) revealed that nurses working in low-dependency forensic wards did not use any formal assessment tools, but that all relied on factors identified in the research as likely indicators of risk.

Actuarial risk assessment has also been criticized as being less sensitive than clinical risk assessment to individual differences since actuarial tools are developed from data on large populations and are therefore not specific to the individual person. Risk at the individual level needs to be assessed using a full clinical

Table 13.2

Examples of risk assessment tools used to predict suicide and self-harm

Name of tool	Additional information	Reference
Suicidal Intent Scale (SIS)	Provides a measure of suicidal intent and lethality of attempts	(Beck et al., 1975)
Scale for Suicide Ideation (SSI)	19-item structured clinical interview and rating scale for measuring suicidality among persons who have recently attempted suicide	(Beck et al., 1979)
Risk-Rescue Rating Scale	Enables evaluation of lethality through assessment of risk-rescue factors	(Weisman & Worden, 1972)
Index of Potential Suicide (IPS)	Two-part schedule with 69 variables	(Zung, 1971)
Neuropsychiatric Hospital Suicide Prevention Schedule	11-item clinician-administered scale	(Farberow & MacKinnon, 1974)
Beck Depression Inventory (BDI)	21-item self-report questionnaire of depressive symptoms	(Beck et al., 1961; Beck & Steer, 1987)
Nurses' Observation Scale for Inpatient Evaluation (NOSIE)	Contains several items concerning identifying active psychotic symptoms	(Honigfeld, 1976)
Beck Hopelessness Scale (BHS)	20-item self-report questionnaire focusing on the construct of hopelessness	(Beck et al., 1974)
Risk Estimator for Suicide	15-item clinician-administered scale	(Motto et al., 1985)
Harkavy-Asnis Suicide Survey (HASS)	A self-report survey	(Harkavy-Friedman & Asnis, 1989)
Modified Scale for Suicidal Ideation (MSSI)	18-item modified version of the SSI	(Joiner et al., 1997)
Problem Solving Inventory (PSI)	32-item self-report measure of problem-solving behaviours and attitudes	(Heppner, 1988)
Life Experiences Survey (LES)	57-item self-report scale focusing on the occurrence of life stress	(Sarason et al., 1978)

assessment of mental state, behaviour and a review of the history. However, an actuarial or statistical approach to risk assessment can enhance the predictions based on clinical assessments and can communicate the degree of risk in quantitative terms. Actuarial risk assessments cannot take the place of clinical assessments, but actuarial data can significantly inform and guide clinical assessments, particularly to avoid underassessments of risk and serious false negatives. The most comprehensive form of risk assessment combines clinical judgement, risk factor identification and the use of actuarial instruments.

Hall (1988) suggests that clinicians should take careful note of available actuarial data when assessing 'dangerousness'. The findings from this study showed that actuarial variables were significantly predictive of sexual reoffences against adults and of non-sexual violent and non-violent reoffending. The author concluded that although the blanket adoption of statistical approaches over clinical approaches is undesirable in the prediction of low-probability events that may have serious consequences, actuarial techniques may help clinicians avoid false negatives.

Similarly, Litwack et al. (1993) suggest that clinicians should think twice about releasing a person predicted to recidivate by the actuarial equation. They suggest that the most useful function of actuarial schemes in the assessment of violent behaviour is to provide a check on clinical judgement. Swett & Mills (1997) evaluated the use of a number of tools for predicting assaults among acutely psychiatrically-ill hospital patients. They found that the tools provided a reasonably accurate way of predicting assaults in the inpatient setting and gave accurate predictions of assault or non-assault 81% of the time.

In relation to suicide assessment, Thienhaus & Piasecki (1997) suggest that rating scales are useful in prompting the necessary inquiries for a complete assessment, but that they cannot and must not replace individual clinical judgement about a particular person's suicide risk. Pokorny (1983), in a large prospective study involving 4800 psychiatric inpatients, found that despite using a number of different suicide risk assessment instruments, attempts to identify people who committed suicide were unsuccessful. Many cases were missed and there were far too many false positives with each of the instruments.

Clark (1990), commenting on studies examining the standardized prediction of suicide, concludes that the realities of low population base rates of completed suicide and the inevitable error rates associated with the best clinical instruments available combine to produce high *false-positive* and high *false-negative* rates, rendering prediction formulae clinically unfeasible under the best of circumstances. In their meta-analysis covering 81 published articles comprising nearly 15,000 subjects, van Egmond & Diekstra (1990) concluded that suicide prediction research had made little headway since the 1960s. Some of the difficulties in this area of research are that there is poor consensus on definitions for suicide, suicide attempt, parasuicide, suicidal ideation and tendency and the validity of the designs is often questionable. Another difficulty with suicide research is that the person committing suicide is no longer there to provide information!

Clinicians may be under pressure to complete their risk assessment so quickly that there is not enough time to complete actuarial assessments (Holloway, 1997). However, one can argue that in a pressured crisis situation an 'objective' tool may be particularly useful for assessing the potential risk.

Lipsedge (1995) suggests that the predictive power of decisions based on actuarial data can be substantially increased by using realistic time frames, which are not too long. This author also suggests that other factors need to be taken into account, such as the environment into which the person is discharged, the person's declared intentions and attitudes to previous and potential new victims, the person's mental state, their ability to take responsibility for their behaviour and to cope with stress. One difficulty in utilizing actuarial data within individual clinical risk assessment is knowing which factors are particularly relevant in the individual case.

CONCLUSION

In this chapter we have highlighted the role that assessing risks and associated crises plays in modern mental health nursing practice. Both clinical and actuarial methods of risk assessment are helpful in giving indications about what may occur in the future. Nevertheless, such methods cannot stand alone in determining what interventions a nurse may agree with a service user and other clinicians. Knowledge of relevant factors that increase a given risk should also be important in helping to focus the nurse's thinking (see Fig. 13.1).

In addition, awareness of factors that impact on the decision-making processes of the nurse (and colleagues) can help to eliminate biases that reduce the accuracy of a risk prediction. We would advocate that mental health nurses do not adhere to a single method or theoretical position when undertaking risk assessment work. Instead, we would urge that nurses obtain as much information as possible in the time allowed to make decisions that can be regarded as objective at that point in time, even if hindsight should prove otherwise.

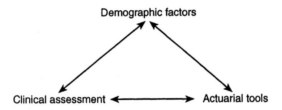

Figure 13.1

Comprehensive risk assessment.

REFERENCES

Addad, M., Benezech, M., Bourgeois, M. & Yesevage, J. (1988) Criminal acts among schizophrenics in French mental hospitals. *Journal of Nervous and Mental Disorders.* 169, 289–293.

Alberg, C., Hatfield, B. & Huxley, P. (1996) *Learning Materials on Mental Health Risk Assessment.* Manchester: Manchester University and Department of Health.

Appleby, L. (1997) Assessment of suicide risk. *Psychiatric Bulletin.* 21, 193–194.

Barratt, E.S. (1994) Impulsiveness and aggression. In: J. Monahan & H.J. Steadman (eds) *Violence and Mental Disorder.* Chicago: University of Chicago Press, pp. 61–79.

Beck, A.T. & Steer, R.A. (1987) *Manual for Beck Depression Inventory.* San Antonio, Texas: Psychological Corporation.

Beck, A.T. & Weishaar, M. E. (1990) Suicide risk assessment and prediction. *Crisis.* 11:2, 22–30.

Beck, A.T., Ward, C.H., Mendelson, M., Mock, J. & Erbaugh, J. (1961) An inventory for measuring depression. *Archives of General Psychiatry.* 4, 561–571.

Beck, A.T., Weissman, A., Lester, D. & Trexler, L. (1974) the measurement of pessimism: The Hopelessness Scale. *Journal of Consulting and Clinical Psychology.* 42, 861–865.

Beck, A.T., Beck, R. & Kovacs, M. (1975) Classification of suicidal behaviours. I: Quantifying intent and medical lethality. *American Journal of Psychiatry.* 132, 285–287.

Beck, A.T., Kovacs, M. & Weissman, A. (1979) An assessment of suicidal intention: the scale for suicide ideation. *Journal of Consulting and Clinical Psychology.* 47:2, 343–352.

Buss, A. & Durkee, A. (1957) An inventory for assessing different kinds of hostility. *Journal of Counselling Psychology.* 21, 342–349.

Clark, D.C. (1990) Suicide risk assessment and prediction in the 1990's. *Crisis.* 11:2, 104–112.

Department of Health (1996) *Building Bridges: A Guide to Arrangements for Interagency Working for Care and Protection of Severely Mentally Ill People.* London: The Stationery Office.

Dohrenwend, B.P., Shrout, B., Link, B., Martin, J. & Skodal, A. (1986) Overview and initial results from a risk factor study of depression and schizophrenia. In: J. E. Barret and R. M. Rose (eds) *Mental Disorders in the Community.* New York: Guilford, pp. 184–215.

Duffy, D. (1993) Preventing suicide. *Nursing Times.* 89:31, 28–30.

Farberow, N.L. & MacKinnon, D. (1974) A suicide prediction schedule for neuropsychiatric hospital patients. *Journal of Nervous and Mental Disease.* 158:6, 408–419.

Folstein, M.F., Folstein, S.E., McHugh, P.R. (1975) Mini-mental state: a practical method for grading the cognitive state of patients for the clinician. *Journal of Psychiatric Research.* 12, 189–198.

Goldcare, M., Seagrott, V. & Hawton, K. (1993) Suicide after discharge from psychiatric care. *Lancet.* 342: 283–286.

Goldstein, R.B., Nasrallah, A. & Winkur, G. (1991) The prediction of suicide. *Archives of General Psychiatry.* 48: 418–422.

Gunn, J. (1993) Dangerousness. In: J. Gunn & P.J. Taylor (eds) *Forensic Psychiatry.* Oxford: Butterworth-Heinemann, pp. 826–828.

Hall, G.C.N. (1988) Criminal behaviour as a function of clinical and actuarial variables in a sexual offender population. *Journal of Consulting and Clinical Psychology.* 56:5, 773–775.

Harkavy-Friedman, J.M. & Asnis, G.M. (1989) Assessment of suicidal behaviour: a new instrument. *Psychiatric Annals.* 19, 382–387.

Hart, S.D., Hare, R.D. & Forth, A.E. (1994) Psychopathy as a risk marker for violence: development and validation of a screening version of the Revised Psychopathy Checklist. In: J. Monahan & H.J. Steadman (eds) *Violence and Mental Disorder.* Chicago: University of Chicago Press, pp. 81–98.

Hawton, K. (1987) Assessment of suicide risk. *British Journal of Psychiatry.* 150, 145–153.

Heppner, P. (1988) *Manual for Problem-Solving Inventory.* Palo Alto, California: Consulting Psychologists Press.

Holloway, F. (1997) The assessment and management of risk in psychiatry: can we do better? *Psychiatric Bulletin.* 21, 283–285.

Honigfeld, G. (1976) NOSIE: Nurses' Observational Scale for Inpatient Evaluation. In: G. Honigfeld (ed) *ECDEU Assessment Manual for Psychopharmacology.* Rockville, Maryland: National Institute of Mental Health, pp. 65–71.

Hughes, D.H. (1996) Suicide and violence assessment in psychiatry. *General Hospital Psychiatry.* 18, 416–421.

Hughes, S.L. &. Neimeyer, R.A. (1993) Cognitive predictors of suicide risk among hospitalized psychiatric patients: a prospective study. *Death Studies.* 17, 103–124.

Hughes, T. & Owen, D. (1996) Management of suicidal risk. *British Journal of Hospital Medicine.* 56:4, 151–154.

Humphreys, M.S., Johnstone, E.C., MacMillan, J.F. & Taylor, P.J. (1992) Dangerous behaviour preceding first admissions for schizophrenia. *British Journal of Psychiatry.* 161, 501–505.

Johnson, J. & Adams, J. (1996) Self-neglect in later life. *Health and Social Care in the Community.* 4:4, 226–233.

Joiner, T.E., Rudd, M. D. & Rajab, M.H. (1997) The Modified Scale for Suicidal Ideation: factors of suicidality and their relation to clinical and diagnostic variables. *Journal of Abnormal Psychology.* 106:2, 260–265.

King, E. (1994) Suicide and the mentally ill: an epidemiological sample and implications for clinicians. *British Journal of Psychiatry.* 165, 658–663.

Krakowski-Jaeger, J. & Volavka, J. (1988) Violence and psychopathology: a longitudinal study. *Comprehensive Psychiatry.* 29, 275–292.

Lidz, C.W., Mulvey, E.P. & Gardner, W. (1993) The accuracy of predictions of violence to others. *Journal of the American Medical Association.* 269:8, 1007–1011.

Limandri, B.J. & Sheridan, D.J. (1995) Prediction of intentional interpersonal violence: An introduction. In: J.C. Campbell (ed) *Assessing Dangerousness: Violence by sexual offenders, batterers and child abusers.* London: Sage. pp. 1–19.

Lindqvist, P. & Allebeck, P. (1990) Schizophrenia and crime. *British Journal of Psychiatry.* 157, 345–350.

Link, B. & Stueve, A. (1994) Psychotic symptoms and the violent/illegal behaviour of mental patients compared to community controls. In: J. Monahan & H.J. Steadman (eds) *Violence and Mental Disorder.* Chicago: University of Chicago Press, pp. 137–159.

Link, B., Andrews, J. & Cullen, F. (1992) The violent and illegal behaviour of mental patients reconsidered. *American Sociological Review.* 57, 275–292.

Lipsedge, M. (1995) Clinical risk management in psychiatry. *Quality in Health Care,* 4, 122–128.

Litwack, T.R., Kirschner, S.M., & Wack, R.C. (1993) The assessment of dangerousness and predictions of violence: recent research and future prospects. *Psychiatric Quarterly.* 64:3, 245–271.

Maiuro, R.D., Vitaliano, P.P. & Cahn, T.S. (1987) A brief measure for the assessment of anger and aggression. *Journal of Interpersonal Violence.* 2, 166–178.

Malone, K.M., Szanto, K., Corbitt, E.M. & Mann, J. J. (1995) Clinical assessment versus research methods in the assessment of suicidal behaviour. *American Journal of Psychiatry.* 152:11, 1601–1607.

Maltsberger, J.T. & Rosenberg, M.L.(1990) The interface between empirical suicide research and clinical practice. *Crisis.* 11:2, 3–10.

McNeil, D.E., & Binder, R.L. (1991) Clinical assessment of the risk of violence among psychiatric inpatients. *American Journal of Psychiatry.* 148:10, 1317–1321.

Miller, M. & Morris, N. (1988) Predictions of dangerousness: an argument for limited use. *Violence and Victims.* 3, 263–284.

Monahan, J. (1981) *Predicting Violent Behaviour: An Assessment of Clinical Techniques.* Beverly Hills, California: Sage.

Monahan, J. (1988) Risk assessment of violence among the mentally disordered: generating useful knowledge. *International Journal of Law and Psychiatry.* 11, 249–257.

Monahan, J. (1992) Mental disorder and violent behaviour: perceptions and evidence. *American Psychologist.* 47:4, 511–521.

Monahan, J. & Steadman, H.J. (1994) Toward a rejuvenation of risk assessment research. In: J. Monahan & H.J. Steadman (eds) *Violence and Mental Disorder.* Chicago: University of Chicago Press, pp. 1–17.

Morgan, H.G. (1997) Management of suicide risk. *Psychiatric Bulletin.* 21, 214–216.

Morgan, H.G. & Priest, P. (1991) Suicide and other unexpected deaths among psychiatric patients. *British Medical Journal.* 158, 368–374.

Mossman, D. (1994) Assessing predictions of violence: being accurate about accuracy. *Journal of Consulting Psychology.* 62:4, 783–792.

Motto, J.A., Heilbron, D.C. & Juster, R.P. (1985) Development of a clinical instrument to estimate suicide risk. *American Journal of Psychiatry.* 142:6, 680–686.

Mullen, P. (1997) Assessing risk of interpersonal violence in the mentally ill. *Advances in Psychiatric Treatment.* 3, 166–173.

Nobel, P. & Rodger, S. (1989) Violence by psychiatric inpatients. *British Journal of Psychiatry.* 155, 384–390.

Novaco, R.W. (1975) *Anger Control: The Development and Evaluation of an Experimental Treatment.* Lexington, Massachusetts: D.C. Heath.

Novaco, R.W. (1994) Anger as a risk factor for violence among the mentally disordered. In: J. Monahan & H.J. Steadman. *Violence and Mental Disorder.* Chicago: University of Chicago Press. pp. 21–59.

Overall, J. & Goreham, D. (1962) The Brief Psychiatric Rating Scale. *Psychology Reports.* 22, 788–812.

Pilgrim, D. & Rogers, A. (1996) Two notions of risk in mental health debates. In: T. Heller, J. Reynolds, R. Gomm, R. Muston & S. Pattison (eds) *Mental Health Matters.* Basingstoke: Macmillan/Open University, pp. 181–185.

Pokorny, A.D. (1983) Prediction of suicide in psychiatric patients. *Archives of General Psychiatry.* 40, 249–257.

Quinsey, V. & Maguire, A. (1979) Variables affecting psychiatrists' and teachers' assessments of the dangerousness of mentally ill offenders. *Journal of Consulting Psychology.* 47:2, 353–362.

Quinsey, V. & Maguire. A. (1986) Maximum security psychiatric patients: actuarial and clinical predictions of dangerousness. *Journal of Interpersonal Violence.* 1:2 143–171.

Reed, P.G. & Leonard, V.E. (1989) An analysis of the concept of self-neglect. *Advances in Nursing Science.* 12:1, 39–53.

Ryan, T. (1996) Risk management and people with mental health problems. In: H. Kemshall & J. Pritchard (eds) *Good Practice in Risk Assessment and Risk Management,* Volume 1. London: Jessica Kingsley Publications, pp. 93–108.

Ryan, T. (1998) Perceived risks associated with mental illness: beyond homicide and suicide. *Social Science and Medicine.* 46:2, 287–297.

Sarason, I., Johnson, J. & Siegel, J. (1978) Assessing the impact of life changes:

development of the Life Experiences Survey. *Journal of Consulting and Clinical Psychology.* 46, 932–946.

Selzer, M. (1971) The Michigan Alcoholism Screening Test: the quest for a new diagnostic instrument. *American Journal of Psychiatry.* 127, 1653–1658.

Skinner, H.A. (1982) The Drug Abuse Screening Test. *Addictive Behaviour.* 7, 363–371.

Spielberger, C.D., Krasner, S.S. & Solomon, E.P. (1988) The experience, expression and control of anger. In: M.P. Janisse (ed) *Health Psychology: Individual Differences and Stress.* New York: Springer Verlag, pp. 89–108.

Swanson, J.W. (1994) Mental disorder, substance abuse and community violence: an epidemiological approach. In: J. Monahan & H.J. Steadman (eds) *Violence and Mental Disorder.* Chicago: University of Chicago Press, pp. 101–136.

Swett, C. & Mills, T. (1997) Use of the NOSIE to predict assaults among acute psychiatric patients. *Psychiatric Services.* 48:9, 1177–1181.

Tan, M.W. & McDonough, W.J. (1990) Risk management in psychiatry. *Psychiatric Clinics of North America.* 13, 135–147.

Taylor, P.J. (1985) Motives for offending among violent and psychotic men. *British Journal of Psychiatry.* 147, 491–498.

Taylor, P.J., Garety, P., Buchanan, A. *et al.* (1994) Delusions and violence. In: J. Monahan & H.J. Steadman (eds) *Violence and Mental Disorder.* Chicago, University of Chicago Press, pp. 161–182.

Thienhaus, O.J. & Piasecki, M. (1997) Assessment of suicide risk. *Psychiatric Services.* 48:3, 293–294.

van Egmond, M. & Diekstra, R.F.W. (1990) The predictability of suicidal behaviour. *Crisis.* 11, 57–84.

Vinestock, M.D. (1996) Risk assessment. A word to the wise? *Advances in Psychiatric Treatment.* 2, 3–10.

Weisman, J.W. & Worden, J.W. (1972) Risk-rescue rating in suicide assessment. *Archives of General Psychiatry.* 26:6, 553–560.

Werner, P.D., Rose, T.L. & Yesavage, J.A. (1990) Aspects of consensus in clinical predictions of imminent violence. *Journal of Clinical Psychology.* 46:4, 534–538.

Wessely, S. (1997) The epidemiology of crime, violence and schizophrenia. *British Journal of Psychiatry.* 170 (supplement 32), 8–11.

Williams, R. & Morgan, G. (eds) (1994) *Suicide Prevention: The Challenge Confronted.* London: HMSO.

Woods, P. (1996) How nurses make assessments of patient dangerousness. *Mental Health Nursing.* 16:4, 20–22.

Yudofsky, S.C., Silver, J.M., Jackson, W., Endicott, J. & Williams, D. (1986) The Overt Aggression Scale for the objective rating of verbal and physical aggression. *American Journal of Psychiatry.* 143, 35–39.

Zung, W.W.K. (1971). Index of potential suicide (IPS). Workshop on the prediction of suicidal behaviour. Philadelphia: National Institute of Mental Health Studies for Suicide Prevention.

£21.50